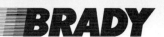BRADY

FIRST AID
IN THE WORKPLACE

WHAT TO DO IN THE FIRST FIVE MINUTES

Second Edition

GRANT B. GOOLD, MPA/HSA, EMT-P

PRENTICE HALL, UPPER SADDLE RIVER, NEW JERSEY 07458

Library of Congress Cataloging-in-Publication Data

Goold, Grant B.
    First aid in the workplace: what to do in the first five minutes
/ Grant B. Goold.—2nd ed.
        p.   cm.
    Includes index.
    ISBN 0-8359-5109-X
    1. First aid in illness and injury—Handbooks, manuals, etc.
2. CPR (First aid)—Handbooks, manuals, etc.   3. Industrial safety—
Handbooks, manuals, etc.   I. Title
    RC86.8.G66   1998   97-12174
    616.02'52—dc21   CIP

Publisher: Susan Katz
Managing development editor: Lois Berlowitz
Project editor: Carole Anderson Lucia
Editorial/production supervision: Janet McGillicuddy
Managing production editor: Patrick Walsh
Director of production/manufacturing: Bruce Johnson
Prepress/manufacturing buyer: Ilene Sanford
Editorial assistant: Carol Sobel
Electronic page make-up: Janet McGillicuddy
Creative Director: Marianne Frasco
Interior design: Claudia Durell
Cover design: Bruce Kenselaar
Interior photographer: John Moore, Marc Longwood, Inc.,
    and Robin Smith

Printed in the United States of America
10   9   8   7   6   5   4   3   2

ISBN 0-8359-5109-X

Prentice-Hall International (UK) Limited, *London*
Prentice-Hall of Australia Pty. Limited, *Sydney*
Prentice-Hall Canada Inc., *Toronto*
Prentice-Hall Hispanoamericana, S.A., *Mexico*
Prentice-Hall of India Private Limited, *New Delhi*
Prentice-Hall of Japan, Inc., *Tokyo*
Pearson Education Asia Pte. Ltd., *Singapore*
Editora Prentice-Hall do Brasil, Ltda., *Rio de Janeiro*

THIS BOOK IS DEDICATED TO EVERY GOOD
SAMARITAN WHO IS WILLING TO HELP OTHERS DURING
TIMES OF CRISIS AND VULNERABILITY

CONTENTS

P R E F A C E

When *First Aid in the Workplace: What to Do in the First Five Minutes* was first published three years ago, it changed the way many people viewed first aid training. Rather than seeing first aid training as a strict, structured, and complicated experience, students who used this program realized just how simple first aid skills are to learn, remember, and perform. Through a revolutionary combination of icons (I call them universal symbols), artwork, and simple writing, students learned first aid skills faster, performed them better, and remembered them longer than when using other first aid texts.

In an effort to provide you with an even better book, I have made a few changes to the second edition of *First Aid in the Workplace: What to Do in the First Five Minutes*. First, I incorporated many recommendations from both students and instructors. Those changes include new and updated information about emergency care for infants and children, training in soft-tissue injury management, and a brief discussion of automated external defibrillation. Thanks to all of you for your suggestions.

Second, I added new material in response to changes in medical standards for first aid responders.

Finally, I included new material based on a document titled "National Guidelines for First Aid Training in Occupational Settings." These guidelines were published and reviewed by leaders in industrial and community first aid training. They are intended to establish national standards regarding the skills that first aid training should encompass.

I strived to sift through the mountain of available material and present only what I believe is necessary to manage almost any emergency situation until professional help arrives. You will therefore not find information on obscure emergencies that you'll likely see only on television. Your instructor can offer additional information about various emergencies as needed. I have also attempted to remove as much medical terminology as possible. That is admittedly not an easy task for a paramedic and emergency medical services educator. Hard as I might have tried to eliminate the jargon, I am sure there are a few remaining terms that I just could not bring myself to part with. Forgive me.

Similar to the first edition of this book, Part 1 of this edition of *First Aid in the Workplace: What to Do in the First Five Minutes* focuses on the universal symbols and their corresponding skills. Only those skills you are most likely to need in an emergency are included. The symbols are presented in the order in which their corresponding skills are typically used in emergency situations. As you progress through the book, each symbol and skill builds on the knowledge you have already gained. As you master the hands-on skills associated with each symbol, you will increase your confidence and willingness to deliver first aid.

Once you are comfortable with the skills presented in Part 1, you are ready to proceed to Part 2. Part 2 includes treatment of those illnesses and injuries most commonly encountered in occupational settings. Your instructor will focus on the chapters in Part 2 that are most applicable to your workplace. Be sure to ask plenty of questions as you progress through this course.

My primary goal in writing this book is to simplify first aid education and increase the number of citizens trained to save lives. Thanks for joining the team. Be safe, and good luck!

Grant B. Goold

ACKNOWLEDGMENTS

I extend gratitude to the following people who assisted me, some directly and others indirectly, in the development of this text program.

Shelley Goold
Marshall & Whitney Meager
Jon Burgess
Lisa Dubnoff
Thom Hillson
American River College
Brent Q. Hafen
Susan Katz
Carole Anderson Lucia
Judy Streger
Carol Sobel
Judy Stamm
John Moore Photography

Carol Bonefield
Reed & Marcia Johnson
Jim Van Brunt
Mark & Angie Bassett
Goold Kids
Blaine Boden
Keith Karren
Lois Berlowitz
Janet McGillicuddy
Patrick Walsh
Image Perspectives
Robin Smith Photography
Marc Longwood, Inc.

I would also like to thank the following reviewers for their comments and suggestions for the revision of this text.

Marty Casarona, BS, EMT-P, CIC
Casarona Training Consultants
Lake Grove, New York

Joey E. Crumby, EMT-P
EMS Concepts of Tennessee
Bolivar, Tennessee

Darrell W. Duty
Mesa Community College
Mesa, Arizona

Paul Hemsley
Omaha First Aid Training Ctr., Inc.
Omaha, Nebraska

Patty Reger, RN
RESA VII
Fairmont, West Virginia

Ham Robbins
Rent-A-Medic
Education Services
Redfield, Maine

Michael K. van Hoek, EMT-P
EMS Training Coordinator
Hillsborough County Fire Rescue
Tampa, Florida

ABOUT THE AUTHOR

Grant B. Goold is Program Director of the EMS Education Center
at American River College in Sacramento. He is also president of
Safety Consultants and is a managing partner of ClasTrak
Software Company.

Grant holds Master's degrees in Public Administration and
Health Services Administration. He is currently in the final year
of his doctoral program in Education/Curriculum and
Instruction at the University of San Francisco. He began his EMS
career in 1985 and continues to work as a field paramedic. Grant
encourages comments about his ideas and concepts.

ROLES AND RESPONSIBILITIES OF FIRST AID RESPONDERS

As a first aid responder, your job description and responsibilities will likely depend to a certain extent on your occupational setting. A few roles do, however, remain constant regardless of your workplace. For example, as a first aid responder, you are always responsible for the following:

- Maintaining your own health and safety.

- Maintaining a professional appearance.

- Maintaining a caring attitude toward your patients, your patients' family members, and bystanders.

- Maintaining your composure and helping others stay calm during medical emergencies.

- Making patients' needs a high priority.

- Keeping your skills and knowledge of emergency first aid up-to-date by attending refresher training courses and continuing education programs.

- Maintaining your knowledge of local, state, and national issues affecting emergency first aid.

This list represents only your most basic responsibilities as a first aid responder. While all of these roles are important, there are many more. Within each of the following chapters, you will learn additional roles, responsibilities, skills, and knowledge that you will need to work most effectively as a first aid responder. (For a complete list of the roles and responsibilities expected of you specifically, contact your organization or local emergency medical services [EMS] agency.)

Your ability to manage a medical response will improve as you progress through this training program. To help you remember the specifics of your roles and responsibilities, make a list, and add to it each time you learn something new. Review this list often, and quiz your fellow students about the various items on it.

MEDICAL EMERGENCY RESPONSE TEAMS

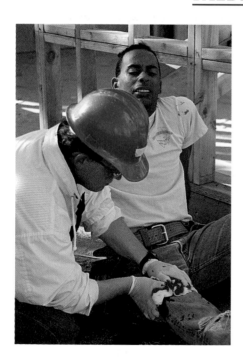

In many organizations, a medical emergency response team (MERT) is the first line of defense in emergencies. MERTs are often found in large organizations or those operating in a potentially hazardous atmosphere, such as chemical companies.

As a member of a MERT, you might be trained in the following areas:

- Use of the various types of fire extinguishers.

- First aid, including *cardiopulmonary resuscitation* (CPR).

- Lockdown-tagout procedures, including machinery and power shutdown.

- Chemical-spill control procedures.

- Use of self-contained breathing apparatus.

- Search and rescue techniques.

- Firefighting.

- Trauma counseling.

As a MERT member, your level of training and response will depend on many factors. Those include your organization's risk and frequency of injuries, the proximity of EMS professionals, and the distance between the organization and nearest medical facility.

BARRIERS TO ACTION

As you know, emergency situations are going to happen. People will occasionally need immediate lifesaving assistance. As a first aid responder, you must quickly and safely identify an emergency and begin delivering competent patient care immediately. Anything less places patients at risk for additional injury or even death.

Research has shown that people who do not feel confident about helping in an emergency are less likely to even acknowledge that an emergency exists. This type of psychological response is known as a *barrier to action*. Other barriers to action include a fear of blood, a fear of injuring the patient, and a fear of liability.

All emergency response personnel must learn to identify and overcome their own barriers to action. You are no different. To help you overcome your personal barriers to action, it can be helpful to talk to experienced first aid responders about how they handle theirs.

As a first aid responder, you must commit to action well in advance of an emergency situation. Why don't you make that commitment to yourself and those around you right now? Commit to the idea of being willing and able to provide lifesaving first aid. Jump right in. Do not hesitate. Be the real hero in your workplace and community.

PATIENT MANAGEMENT STRATEGIES

Emergency situations come in all sizes, shapes, and colors. Not only is each situation unique, but so are the reactions, complaints, and concerns of patients, family members, co-workers, and bystanders.

Unfortunately, there will be times when the reactions of people around you can distract you from your primary responsibility of delivering patient care. One of the best strategies for maintaining your focus and not allowing yourself to be distracted is to consistently use the same steps in your *initial assessment*, early interventions, and *ongoing assessment*. (We'll discuss these concepts in-depth later in the book.) Letting yourself get caught up in issues that have nothing to do with delivering care to your patient can have potentially negative—if not fatal—consequences.

Another way to manage patients effectively is by designing appropriate emergency action plans. These plans will help you remember the steps necessary to safely, consistently, and competently provide first aid.

In each of the chapters in Section II, you will be encouraged to develop emergency action plans after new material is presented. Practice, refine, and practice again these action plans in preparation for the real thing.

MEDICAL AND ETHICAL ISSUES

Can you imagine being a first aid responder without having received any real medical training or without having someone more experienced oversee the care you deliver? Can you picture the chaos, confusion, and medical liability that would result under such conditions?

To reduce the chances of this occurring, local, state, and national EMS agencies have established standards and regulations defining the skills and actions you can legally perform while delivering first aid. These standards and regulations are collectively known as your *scope of practice*. A system of medical oversight and other processes have also been established to help protect you in your delivery of patient care.

GOOD SAMARITAN

In most states, first aid responders are not legally obligated to provide emergency care. In fact, state law generally protects any voluntary care that first aid responders might provide.

Together, the various rules, policies, regulations, and statutes that protect providers of voluntary first aid are called the *Good Samaritan laws*. These laws help protect you from unfounded legal action that might be taken against you as a result of the patient care you deliver. They will not, however, protect you if your actions were outside your scope of practice or were negligent.

Check with your local EMS agency to determine the specifics of your state's Good Samaritan laws.

CONSENT

All competent adults ultimately have control over what happens to their bodies. As such, you may not provide emergency care to anyone without first obtaining his or her consent. The courts have broken down consent into three specific types:

1. **Expressed consent.** This type of consent is given by a competent adult after being informed of the various steps of the procedure to be performed and their related risks.

2. **Implied consent.** This type of consent is assumed when an unresponsive patient requires emergency intervention.

3. **Children and mentally incompetent adult consent.** This type of consent is obtained from the parent or legal guardian of someone who is incapable of giving expressed or implied consent.

Get into the habit of obtaining consent before you provide any emergency care. Failure to obtain consent prior to delivering treatment could give a patient or guardian grounds for taking legal action against you.

REFUSAL OF CARE

Competent adults can legally refuse all lifesaving care. In fact, many adults have died because they refused to receive such care.

As a first aid responder, you must respect a patient's right to refuse care. If you ever have any questions about a patient's competency or the decisions made for a child or incompetent adult patient, immediately notify your local law enforcement or EMS agency.

ABANDONMENT AND NEGLIGENCE

As a first aid responder, you are accountable for your actions during every emergency situation. If you abandon an ill or injured patient without first delivering appropriate medical care, you could be guilty of abandonment. The best defense against this type of situation is to continue delivering care until someone of greater medical authority, such as an advanced-level EMS responder, assumes medical control of your patient.

Another issue to be aware of is negligence. Despite your best efforts and intentions, you could be accused of negligence. However, four conditions must be proven to have existed before a charge of negligence will stand up in court:

1. You must have had a contractual or legal obligation to deliver care. This is called duty to act.

2. It must be proven that you failed to act or to act appropriately. This is called breach of duty.

3. It must be proven that injury or damages occurred.

4. It must be proven that your actions—or lack of action—directly caused the injury or damages.

CONFIDENTIALITY

The importance of patients' medical information remaining confidential cannot be overstated. Patients could tell you confidential medical information which, if improperly managed, might destroy their professional and personal lives. An example is if a patient tells you that he or she has AIDS.

You must be very careful when dealing with patients' medical information. Never divulge confidential medical information without first having the patient sign a written release. A release is not needed if other health care providers need pertinent medical information about a patient to continue delivering proper emergency care. A release also is not needed if state law requires reporting such information, or if you receive a subpoena requiring that the information be released.

DELIVERING CARE TO INFANTS AND CHILDREN

An increasing number of workplaces now offer on-site day care. In fact, in some occupational settings, infants and children comprise the majority of the population.

For most EMS responders, emergencies involving infants or children present not only a medical challenge but an emotional one as well. If you are asked to care for a sick or injured child, take a few seconds, and do whatever you can to relax. Taking a few deep breaths and reassuring yourself should help you cope with any anxiety you might be feeling.

Beyond practicing some relaxation techniques, the following tips can help when delivering care to an infant or child:

- If one of the child's parents is present and is calm, let him or her help you assess and communicate with the child. If the parent is not calm enough to help, or if the child's injury or illness is severe, ask the parent to stay out of the child's sight. This will help you maintain control of the situation.

- Bend down to the child's level. Towering over a child will only increase his or her anxiety, fear, and unwillingness to cooperate. Speak to the child in a calming tone.

- When treating older children, try to be objective. Do not judge them. Listen!

- Never lie to your patient.

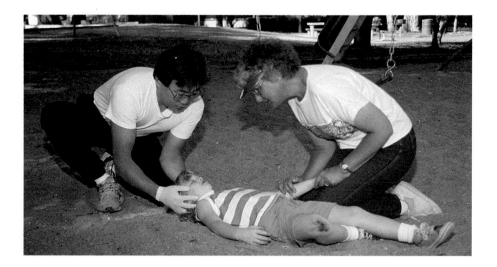

COMMON CHILDHOOD EMERGENCIES

As a first aid responder, you should become familiar with the common illnesses and injuries encountered in infants and children. Perhaps the most common are airway obstructions, respiratory infections, and traumatic accidents.

As most parents will tell you, children will have many bouts with respiratory infections throughout their childhood. *Croup*, which is characterized by a seal-like barking cough, is one such infection. When a child has croup, he or she will have a sore throat, cough, and fever. The onset is generally slow, and the child's symptoms are worse at night. Care includes contacting the child's physician.

Epiglottitis is another respiratory infection. It causes swelling of the throat tissue just above the esophagus. This condition quickly worsens as the tissue begins to close off the airway. Signs of epiglottitis are a sudden high fever, drooling, and an inability to swallow. Epiglottitis is life-threatening. Immediate activation of the EMS system is critical.

Another emergency you may encounter is *sudden infant death syndrome (SIDS)*. Occasionally, seemingly healthy infants die suddenly without warning or known cause. When the reason for death cannot be determined, the death is commonly categorized as SIDS. While SIDS is not necessarily common, it is important to be aware of it. It is one of the most emotionally wrenching situations you could face as a first aid responder.

If you ever have to respond to a possible SIDS situation, it will likely be very difficult for you emotionally. Keep in mind that your professionalism and respect for the family members' emotions will have a major impact on their grieving and healing process. Contact your local EMS agency to determine the protocol for handling SIDS cases.

If you would like to learn more about pediatric illnesses or injuries, contact your local EMS agency for information on pediatric first aid training classes in your area.

STRESS MANAGEMENT

Any experienced EMS responder will tell you that stress is a part of the emergency response experience. But it is not necessarily a good part. Therefore, you must recognize and deal with emergency response stress early and effectively. Refusing to acknowledge destructive stress will only shorten your career as a first aid responder.

Always keep an eye out for these warning signs of stress in yourself as well as your co-workers:

- Irritability toward co-workers, family, and friends.

- An inability to concentrate.

- Nightmares or difficulty sleeping.

- Anxiety.

- Indecisiveness.

- Guilt.

- Loss of appetite.

- Loss of interest in sexual activities.

- Isolation.

- Loss of interest in work.

If you do find that you are suffering from stress, it can be helpful to practice these simple stress-management techniques:

- Reduce the amount of sugar, caffeine, fatty foods, and alcohol you consume. If possible, avoid alcohol altogether.

- Exercise more often.

- Practice relaxation techniques.

- Improve the balance between your family, work, recreation, and health practices.

Dealing with the stress of emergency first aid is a serious issue. You must take responsibility for not only your physical well-being but your mental well-being as well. This could even require calling on mental health professionals to help you cope with a particularly stressful emergency response. Such situations might include an on-the-job death of a co-worker, seriously injured children, or multiple-patient situations.

In these types of situations, mental health professionals might be brought in along with specially trained first aid responders to help you deal with the stress you are experiencing. They often use a practice called *critical incident stress management* or *debriefing*.

Your workplace should be equipped to help you handle any work-related stress you might experience. Never be afraid to share your feelings about any response with members of your first aid responder team.

P A R T 1

UNIVERSAL SYMBOLS TRAINING

Scene Safety

Body Substance Isolation

Activation of EMS

Initial Assessment

Ongoing Assessment

Rescue Breathing and Artificial Ventilation

Cardiopulmonary Resuscitation

Shock

Soft-Tissue Care

Musculoskeletal Care

Spinal Precautions

Oxygen Application

C H A P T E R 1

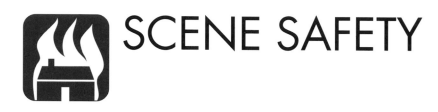 SCENE SAFETY

Before delivering care to any patient, you must take steps to protect your own safety and the safety of other first aid responders. The first way to do this is by evaluating the scene of an emergency and determining if it is safe to enter.

Neglecting to evaluate the scene could put you at risk for becoming a patient yourself. Workplace violence, electrical accidents, toxic spills, fires, floods, auto accidents, collapsed buildings, and explosions are just a few examples of scenes that could be unsafe for you to enter.

After determining that the scene is safe and taking *body substance isolation precautions* (see Chapter 2), you must quickly determine the cause of the patient's accident, injury, or illness. This is done by asking the patient questions that are clear and to the point. If the patient is unconscious or otherwise unable to communicate, question any available bystanders about what happened. Gathering this type of information is known as determining the *mechanism of injury or illness*.

After an accident, a variety of collisions and impacts can take place between organs within the body depending on the mechanism of injury involved. These in turn can cause a number of hidden injuries. As you try to determine the mechanism of injury, think about the forces involved, the body parts affected, and all possible injuries. Once you have this information, you can better estimate potential injuries or problems before they become obvious—or deadly.

STEPS

SCENE SAFETY EVALUATION

1. Obtain as much information as possible about the medical emergency before entering the scene. If there is any possibility of danger, do not enter the scene.

2. If violence is involved, notify your local law enforcement agency, and request assistance.

3. If necessary, communicate with the patient from a safe distance.

4. If you are specially trained to handle dangerous scenes and have the proper *personal protective devices* (see Chapter 2), you may enter the scene and deliver care to the patient.

DANGER

Always take the time to evaluate the scene before you deliver patient care. The one time you forget this life-saving step could very well be your last. With experience, you will begin to trust your instincts. EMS veterans call this their "street sense" or "sixth sense."

C H A P T E R 2

BODY SUBSTANCE ISOLATION

After ensuring that the scene is safe to enter, you must take steps to protect yourself from other potential hazards. This includes protecting yourself from diseases the patient might have and using the proper techniques to lift or move the patient.

Any disease that can be passed from one person to another is called a *communicable,* or *infectious, disease.* There are many infectious diseases that you could come into contact with while delivering patient care. Some common examples are HIV/AIDS and hepatitis, although there are many more. You must take all necessary precautions to prevent yourself from contracting any of them.

As a first aid responder, there are two ways you can become infected with a communicable disease. One way is to become infected by direct contact with blood and other body fluids. It is also possible to become infected by indirect contact. This includes breathing infected airborne droplets from patients with tuberculosis or other respiratory diseases.

Body Substance Isolation Precautions

The best way to protect yourself from contracting communicable diseases is by taking body substance isolation precautions. You must take body substance isolation precautions with **all** patients,

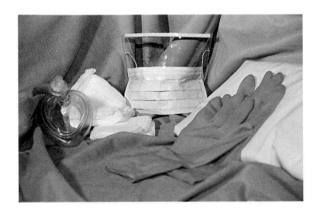

Personal protective devices.

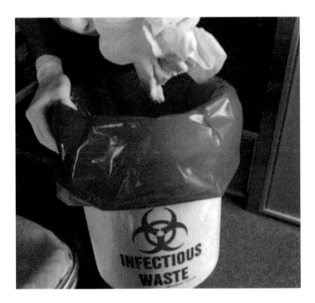

Dispose of all contaminated materials properly.

DANGER

Remember, do not make judgments about patients' disease potential based on the way they look, dress, act, or smell.

regardless of their appearance, the environment they are found in, or their medical problem. This includes using basic common sense, keeping your immunizations up-to-date, and using personal protective devices.

Optimal use of personal protective devices includes using disposable gloves, an eye and face shield, a gown, and a pocket mask. Sometimes using all of these devices is not possible or necessary. In these cases—and when making contact with any patient—you must use gloves and eye protection at the very least.

If disposable gloves are not immediately available and waiting to find some could cause serious harm to the patient, use anything that will not allow blood or other fluids to come into contact with your skin. This might include plastic bags, thick cloth materials, or sturdy leather gloves. (For this reason, it makes good sense to keep several pairs of disposable gloves in your desk, break room, car, and pocket.)

When you are finished delivering care to your patient, keep your gloves on while you gather all of the contaminated materials you used. Then dispose of the materials properly by placing them in the appropriate designated containers. You must never place contaminated materials in standard trash cans. Unsuspecting co-workers could infect themselves.

Once you have gathered the contaminated items and disposed of them, carefully remove your gloves. Take care not to touch the contaminated side of them. Fold each glove into the other as you remove them. Then place them in the same container as the other items. Practice this technique until you can remove every pair of gloves every time without contaminating yourself.

EMERGENCY MOVES AND BACK SAFETY

Using the proper techniques to lift or move the patient is another way you can protect yourself from potential hazards.

In most situations, however, you should not attempt to move the patient. Doing so can cause additional injury. It is better to

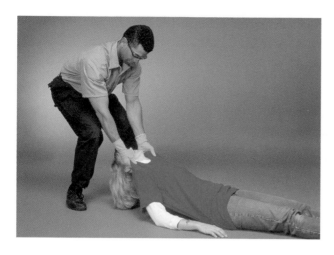

The shirt drag.

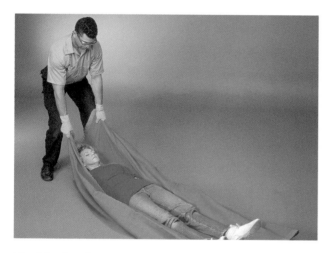

The blanket drag.

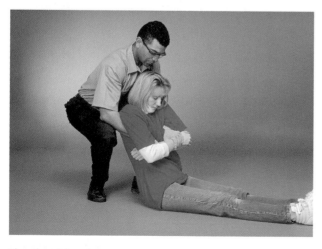

The shoulder drag.

wait for the advanced-level EMS professionals to arrive and move the patient if necessary.

Occasionally, however, you might need to move a patient. This is warranted if you are unable to keep the patient's airway clear so he or she can breathe. Moving a patient is also warranted if he or she is blocking access to other patients who need your help, or if conditions place you or your patient in danger.

If it is necessary to move a patient, use either the shirt drag, blanket drag, or shoulder drag. These emergency moves are designed only to quickly move a patient away from immediate danger. They are not designed to move the patient great distances. Nor are they designed to protect the patient's neck or back from injury.

The shirt drag is performed by grabbing the patient's clothing and pulling him or her in a straight line. The blanket drag is performed essentially the same way, except that the patient is lying on a blanket, piece of carpet, or other large item. The shoulder drag is self-explanatory. Before using the shoulder drag to move a patient, make sure that he or she does not have a serious shoulder injury.

When moving any patient, it is very important that you help protect yourself from back injuries. Back injuries are a serious issue because they can quickly end your career as a first aid responder. Follow these few simple rules to protect yourself when moving any patient:

- Estimate your patient's weight.

- Know your own physical limitations.

- Keep your back locked in a normal, inwardly curved position.

- Use your leg and abdominal muscles to lift—not your back muscles.

- Keep the patient's weight close to your body.

- If other people arc helping you lift a patient, communicate with them throughout the lift. Make sure they know what you are doing and what you expect of them.

- Before you ever get to the point of lifting a patient, work with other team members to develop a safe lifting strategy.

- Perhaps the most important thing you can do before lifting any patient is to ask yourself, "Am I about to do something that could cause me serious injury?" If the answer is yes, stop and get more help.

RECOVERY POSITION

Most patients will be sitting up or lying on their backs as you treat them. In some cases, however, you may need to place a patient in a position that helps protect his or her airway. This is called the *recovery position*. To place a patient in the recovery position, gently roll the patient onto his or her side. As you do this, make sure that the patient's head, shoulders, and torso move together, without twisting.

An example of a patient who should be placed in the recovery position is one who is unconscious, has a pulse, is breathing adequately, and has no signs of trauma or mechanism of injury suggesting serious neck or back trauma.

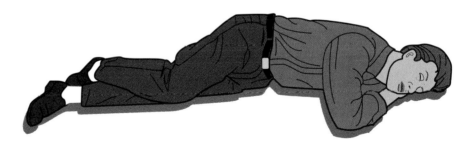

The recovery position.

CHAPTER 3

ACTIVATION OF THE EMERGENCY MEDICAL SERVICES SYSTEM

As a first aid responder, you are a valuable member of the emergency medical services (EMS) system. Other members of the system include firefighters, emergency medical technicians, paramedics, emergency nurses and physicians, and law-enforcement personnel.

The various types of EMS responders have different roles and responsibilities. However, they all work together to provide patients with the best medical care available. As a first aid responder or member of a medical emergency response team, you play perhaps the most important role in any EMS system. You are typically the first person on scene, you are responsible for recognizing that an emergency exists, you know how and when to activate the EMS system, and you can provide basic medical care.

As a first aid responder, you must be able to quickly recognize when the EMS system needs to be activated. Quick activation of the EMS system is a critical step in reducing the number of preventable injuries and deaths. Studies have proven that the earlier you are able to access the EMS system, the quicker the response time and, consequently, the greater the chances of having a positive patient outcome. Don't forget that the sooner the EMS system is activated, the less time you will be required to handle the emergency without other professional help!

THE EMS SYSTEM AT WORK

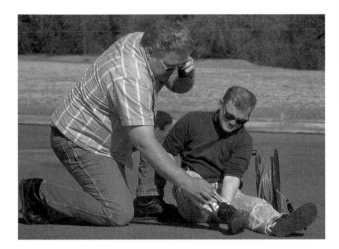

An accident occurs, and the EMS system is activated.

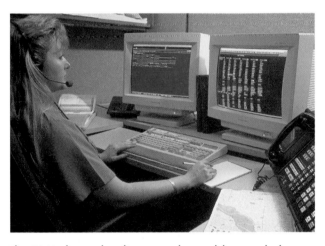

The EMS dispatcher listens to the problem and alerts the appropriate EMS personnel.

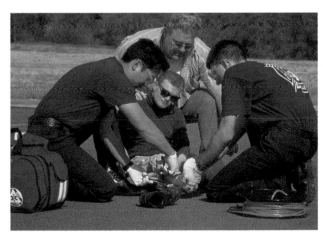

EMS personnel arrive to assess the emergency and deliver care to the patient.

DANGER

Never hang up the phone until you are directed to do so by the emergency medical dispatcher. If you have a portable or cellular phone, take it with you to the patient's side.

In most regions of the country, the EMS system is activated by dialing 9-1-1. In some areas, however, special codes or emergency numbers may be required. Find out now how to activate your EMS system. Then post the appropriate phone numbers in large, bold print next to every phone in your workplace.

Once you have determined that the EMS system should be activated and dialed the appropriate number, you will reach an emergency medical dispatcher. Be prepared to speak clearly and slowly. Quickly answer the dispatcher's questions, and listen carefully to any directions that might be given. EMS personnel will simultaneously be notified as the dispatcher asks questions.

Questions you might be asked include:

- What is the emergency?
- What is your calling location?
- Where is the patient located?
- Is the patient breathing?
- What have you done for the patient?

CHAPTER 4

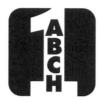 INITIAL ASSESSMENT

Once you have made sure that the scene is safe and taken body substance isolation precautions, you must determine whether the patient is suffering from any life-threatening conditions. If so, you must correct them immediately or as soon as you find them. This is accomplished by doing an initial assessment. Every patient must immediately receive an initial assessment, which should take no longer than 60 seconds to complete.

The initial assessment is undoubtedly the most important series of skills you will learn. It involves checking and managing the basic necessities of life. If these necessities are not managed correctly, your patient can die.

The initial assessment is intended to make sure that the patient's airway is clear, that the patient is breathing adequately, that the patient's circulation is functioning, and that the patient is not suffering from massive bleeding. This is called the *ABCH (airway, breathing, circulation, hemorrhage) assessment process*.

A simple yet complete procedure has been developed to help you learn and perform the initial assessment. As you learn how to do your assessment, you must practice it as often as possible and with as many different people as

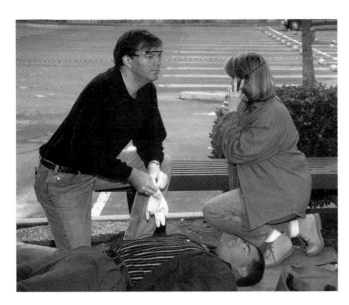

After confirming the safety of the scene, begin to form a general impression of the patient, any potential mechanisms of injury or illness, and the immediate surroundings.

possible. Get into the habit of performing the steps of the initial assessment in exactly the same order each time so you are sure to not omit any steps. Have a friend watch you and take notes on how you are progressing. Make sure that by the end of this program your assessment is flawless and you follow every one of the steps every time.

Before you actually begin assessing your patient, spend a few seconds looking at the immediate surroundings and at the patient to form a general impression of what might have happened. Ask yourself or any bystanders these questions:

- Is this a medical or trauma-related problem?

- What is the patient's approximate age?

- What is the patient's sex?

- Am I going to need assistance from other first aid responders?

- What was done for the patient prior to my arrival?

STEPS

INITIAL ASSESSMENT

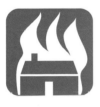

1. Ensure that the scene is safe.

2. Take appropriate body substance isolation precautions.

3. Determine if the patient is responsive by using the shake and shout method. There are four general levels of responsiveness. They are known as the *AVPU scale:*

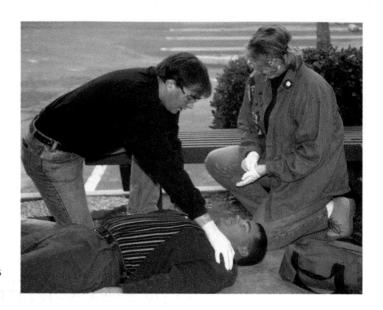

Checking the patient's level of responsiveness using the shake and shout method.

Alert—The patient responds appropriately.

Verbal—The patient responds to verbal stimuli, but not appropriately.

Painful—The patient responds to painful stimuli only, such as a pinched finger.

Unresponsive—The patient is unconscious.

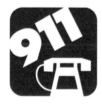 Infants and younger children will not respond to the same methods used to assess responsiveness in adults. You must modify your techniques by rubbing the soles of their feet or blowing in their faces.

 4. If the patient does not respond appropriately or appears to be unconscious, immediately activate the EMS system. If possible, have someone else do this so you can remain with the patient.

5. **A = Airway.** Open the patient's airway using the *head-tilt/chin-lift maneuver*. In cases of suspected neck injuries, use the *jaw-thrust maneuver*.

6. **B = Breathing.** Check to see if the patient is breathing using the *look, listen, and feel* method. Look to see if the patient's chest is rising and falling. Listen for breath sounds from the patient's mouth or nose. Feel for chest movement with your hand and for air against your cheek.

7. If the patient is not breathing, begin *rescue breathing* (see Chapter 6).

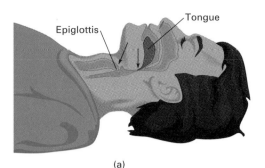
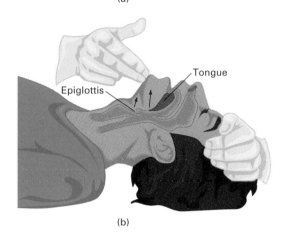

(a)

(b)

The head-tilt/chin-lift maneuver.

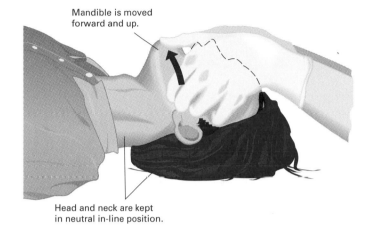

Mandible is moved forward and up.

Head and neck are kept in neutral in-line position.

The jaw-thrust maneuver.

8. **C = Circulation.** Check to see if the patient has a pulse.

- In the responsive adult, assess the *radial* (wrist) *pulse*.

- In the unresponsive adult, assess the *carotid* (neck) *pulse*.

 In the responsive child, assess either the *brachial* (upper arm) or *radial pulse*.

 In the unresponsive child, assess the carotid pulse.

 In any infant, assess the brachial pulse first. If you do not find a brachial pulse, check for a *femoral* (groin) *pulse*.

9. If the patient does not have a pulse, immediately begin *chest compressions* and rescue breathing (see Chapter 7).

10. **H = Hemorrhage.** Quickly run your gloved hands completely over and under the patient, periodically checking your hands for evidence of massive bleeding. If you are in a dark area, have someone quickly get a flashlight for you.

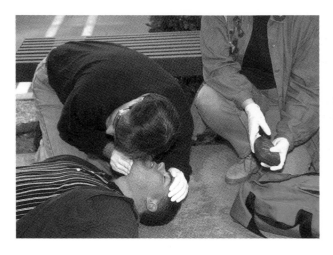

Assessing the airway using the look, listen, and feel method.

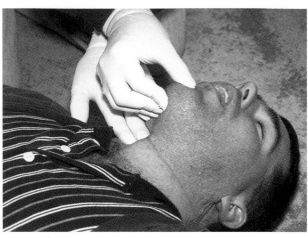

Assessing the patient's carotid pulse.

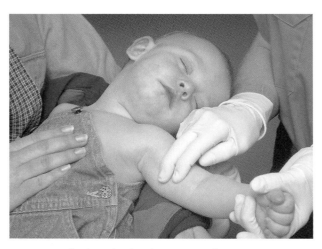

Assessing the brachial pulse in an infant.

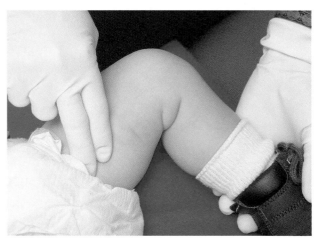

Assessing the femoral pulse in an infant.

11. If the patient is hemorrhaging, control the bleeding by applying direct finger or hand pressure over the wound. If an extremity is involved, elevate the wound and apply hand pressure to the pressure points (see Chapter 9).

TRIAGE

Not all medical emergencies involve only one patient. You may be called on to provide care to several patients at once. This can quickly become problematic if the number of patients is greater than the number of first aid responders.

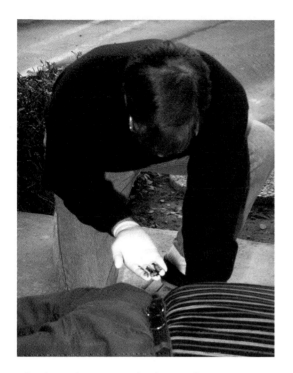

Checking the patient for hemorrhaging.

Based on lessons learned in times of war, a way of prioritizing patients according to the severity of their injuries or illnesses has been developed. This method of patient prioritization is called *triage*. It allows you to provide the best care to the greatest number of people. In some rare cases, triage may dictate that some patients not be treated if their injuries are so severe or so minor that other patients would die if your efforts were directed toward them.

This is a very difficult skill to practice and implement. Contact your local EMS agency to learn how your local triage system works.

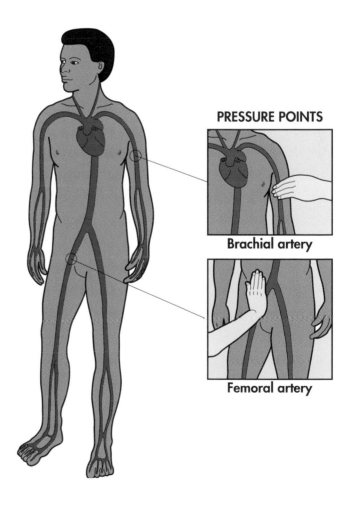

PRESSURE POINTS

Brachial artery

Femoral artery

CHAPTER 5

2 ONGOING ASSESSMENT

Once you have completed an initial assessment of the patient and treated any life-threatening conditions you find, you should perform a head-to-toe physical exam and history. This is also known as an ongoing assessment. This assessment provides additional information about any injuries the patient may have, including their location and severity. In some cases, you might use the ongoing assessment to help determine the patient's main problem, or *chief complaint*, if you weren't able to determine it during the initial assessment.

Under no circumstances should you begin the ongoing assessment if you are unable to control the patient's ABCH. In this case, you must continue to focus on opening the patient's airway, providing *artificial ventilations*, maintaining circulation, and controlling hemorrhaging. These always take priority over the ongoing assessment.

As you do your ongoing assessment, look for medical alert medallions around the patient's ankles, wrist, or neck. These can be good clues as to what might be causing the patient's problem. Other clues can surface as you inspect the patient's body. You may find, however, that you must remove the patient's clothing if it interferes with your assessment or treatment. If you do remove his or her clothing, be sure to do it discreetly.

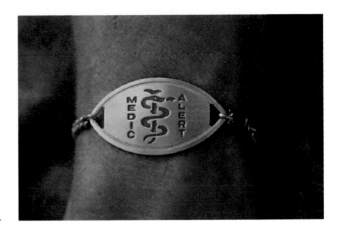

Medical alert medallion.

You must also constantly communicate with the patient while you perform your ongoing assessment. This includes asking questions about the accident and any injuries you might find, and telling the patient what you are doing. In addition to giving you information about the patient's illness or injury, this communication helps you monitor his or her level of consciousness. (Questions specific to different problems will be covered in upcoming chapters.)

As you proceed with your ongoing assessment, you must regularly recheck the patient's ABCH status. In stable patients, the initial assessment should be repeated at least every 15 minutes. In unstable patients, it should be repeated at least every five minutes. If at any time the patient's ABCH status changes, immediately stop your ongoing assessment, perform another initial assessment, and correct any problems you encounter.

During the ongoing assessment, you will look and feel for the following signs of injury:

Deformities

Open injuries

Tenderness

Swelling

Each time you assess an area of your patient's body, you will look and feel for these signs. The mnemonic *DOTS* will help you remember exactly what you are looking for.

 Some infants and children may become agitated if you suddenly start examining their head and face. One technique that often works in these situations is to start at the patient's feet and work your way up the body.

PATIENT HISTORY

As you perform the ongoing assessment, begin asking the patient questions about his or her medical history. In trauma patients, questions can be asked during or after the ongoing assessment. In patients with non-life-threatening medical problems, history questions can be asked before, during, or after the ongoing assessment.

To help focus your questioning, the mnemonic *SAMPLE* works well. SAMPLE stands for:

S = Signs and symptoms. *Signs* are any medical or trauma conditions that the patient **displays**. They can also be any conditions that you identify. *Symptoms* are any conditions that the patient **describes**. To help determine the patient's signs and symptoms, ask, "What is the problem?"

A = Allergies. Allergies can be caused by medication, food, or environmental factors. To find out if the patient has any allergies, ask, "Are you allergic to anything?"

M = Medications. These can be prescription or over-the-counter. To find out if the patient is taking any medications, ask, "Do you take any medications?"

P = Pertinent past history. This can include recent surgery, trauma, or illnesses. To help determine the patient's pertinent past history, ask, "Are you currently seeing a doctor for anything?"

L = Last oral intake. This includes solids and liquids, as well as the quantity consumed. To find out when the patient's last oral intake was, ask, "When was the last time you had anything to eat or drink?"

E = Events leading to the injury or illness. To determine what events could have caused the patient's illness or injury, ask, "What were you doing when this happened?"

As you gather answers to these questions, make sure to have another first aid responder write them down. If you have decided that the EMS system should be activated, this information will be given to the responding EMS crew. Be prepared to tell the responders the following information:

- The patient's age and sex.
- The patient's chief complaint.

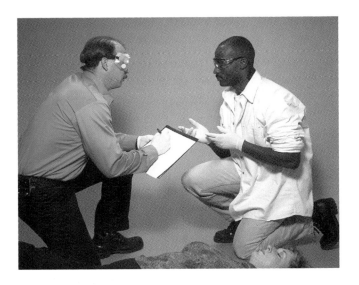

Patient hand-off report to EMS personnel.

- The patient's level of responsiveness, including any changes you have noted.

- The patient's airway and breathing status.

- The patient's circulation status.

- Your ongoing assessment findings.

- The results of your SAMPLE history.

- Any interventions or treatment you provided.

TIME AND TRAUMA

Patients who are suffering from severe trauma have the best chance of survival if they can be delivered to an operating room within one hour of their injuries. This is known as the *golden hour*. To help meet the golden-hour goal, EMS personnel are trained to spend a maximum of 10 minutes on scene with trauma patients.

Because time is such a critical factor in trauma situations, you must quickly recognize the need for EMS and immediately activate the EMS system. Saving time helps save lives!

STEPS

ONGOING ASSESSMENT

1. Ensure that the scene is safe.

2. Take appropriate body substance isolation precautions.

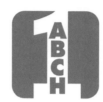

3. Perform an initial assessment.

4. Begin the ongoing assessment by inspecting the patient's head for DOTS.

5. Inspect the patient's neck and shoulders for DOTS.

6. Inspect the patient's chest for DOTS.

7. Inspect the patient's abdomen for DOTS.

8. Inspect the patient's pelvis for DOTS.

9. Inspect the patient's legs for DOTS.

10. Inspect the patient's arms for DOTS.

11. Inspect the patient's back for DOTS—but only if no head or neck injury is suspected.

Make a mental note of any injuries you find. Treat specific injuries after you have

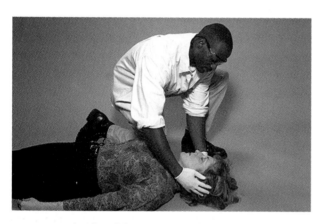

Inspecting the head for DOTS.

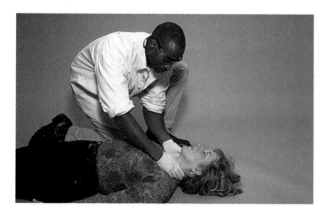

Inspecting the neck for DOTS.

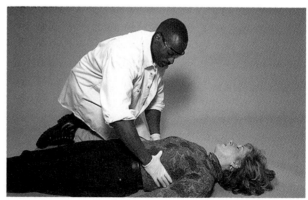

Inspecting the chest for DOTS.

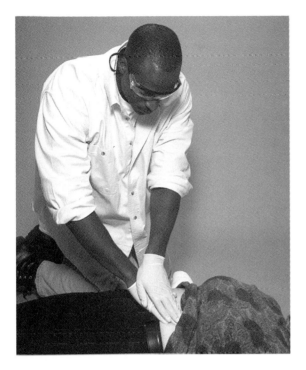

Inspecting the abdomen for DOTS.

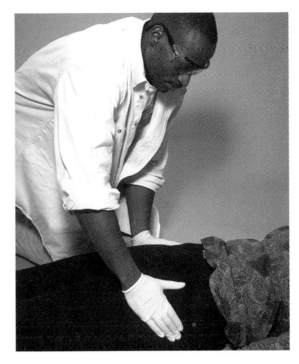

Inspecting the pelvis for DOTS.

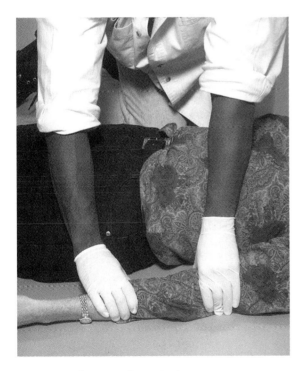

Inspecting the arms for DOTS.

completed your ongoing assessment and properly managed the patient's ABCH.

Do not become alarmed if you are unable to begin or finish your ongoing assessment or SAMPLE history. You may find yourself in emergency situations in which you are only able to maintain the patient's ABCH. But if you do this properly, you have done a good job. Remember that all the information in the world does a patient little good if you neglect to manage his or her airway, breathing, circulation, or hemorrhaging.

DANGER

If a patient is injured, make sure that you move him or her as little as possible. A patient with head or back injuries should be moved only if absolutely necessary, and only by using one of the emergency moves described in Chapter 2.

AIRWAY MANAGEMENT: BASIC LIFE SUPPORT AND ARTIFICIAL VENTILATION

As part of the initial assessment, you will assess and manage the patient's breathing. In most first aid situations, the patient will be able to breathe easily and without any problems. In these cases, you will simply monitor the patient until EMS arrives—if you determine that the EMS system needs to be activated. In rare cases, however, the patient might be breathing very slowly or not at all. In these cases, you need to breathe for the patient.

Adults stop breathing for various reasons. The most common causes are trauma, *cardiac arrest*, drug overdose, stroke, and *foreign-body airway obstructions* (FBAOs), or choking. Infants and children also stop breathing for a number of reasons. The most common causes are FBAOs, trauma, airway diseases, and birth defects.

Regardless of the cause, if a patient is not breathing, you must provide artificial ventilations for him or her. This is also called rescue breathing. The goal of rescue breathing is to fill the patient's lungs with your expired air. This in turn allows lifesaving oxygen to be delivered to the patient's bloodstream.

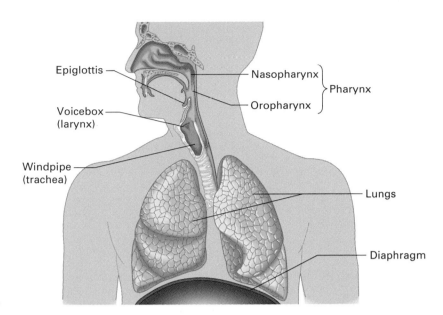

The human respiratory system.

THE HUMAN AIRWAY

The airway is one of the most important parts of the human respiratory system. If it is not kept open and clear, the patient will not be able to breathe. You must therefore closely monitor the airways of all patients and be able to keep them open. This is called *airway management*. When practicing airway management, it is important that you pay close attention to the patient's tongue. It is a critical part of airway management because it is such a large muscle. When the tongue is relaxed or not in its normal position, it can block the airway. This can keep air from passing through the trachea to the lungs.

All airways are not the same. For example, children and adults have the same airway components. Yet the size and strength of

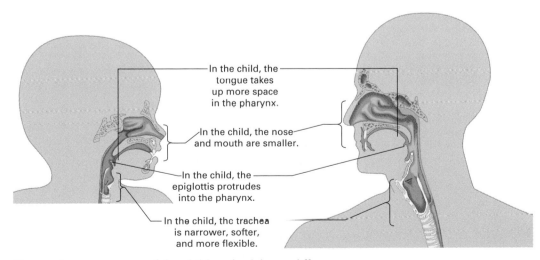

The respiratory systems of the child and adult are different.

each part differs depending on whether it is a child's or adult's. It is important that you realize these differences. Study them carefully. Be prepared to discuss during airway-management skills practice.

STEPS

RESCUE BREATHING

1. Ensure that the scene is safe.

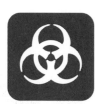

2. Take appropriate body substance isolation precautions.

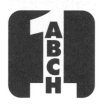

3. Perform part A of the initial assessment. Open and clear the patient's airway. In patients without suspected spine injury, use the head-tilt, chin-lift maneuver. In trauma patients or patients with suspected spine injury, use the jaw-thrust maneuver.

4. Perform part B of the initial assessment. Determine whether the patient is breathing by using the look, listen, and feel method. If the patient isn't breathing or is breathing less than every three to five seconds, you must begin rescue breathing.

5. If you are using mouth-to-mouth, pinch the patient's nose shut. You may omit this step if you are using a pocket mask.

6. Place a pocket mask over the patient's mouth and nose. Be sure to create and maintain a tight seal between the mask and the patient's face. Then place your mouth over the mask's inlet port.

7. Deliver two slow breaths, exhaling into the patient's mouth. Each breath should take approximately 1.5 to 2.0 seconds to deliver. Be sure to watch that the chest rises and falls. This is how you know that your ventilations are being delivered properly. Allow the chest to rise and fall between each breath.

ADULT

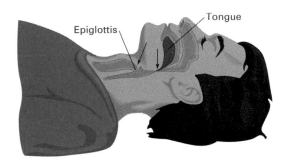

(a)

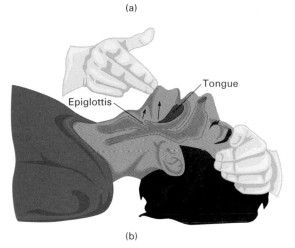

(b)

The head-tilt/chin-lift maneuver.

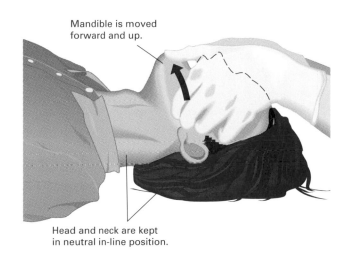

The jaw-thrust maneuver.

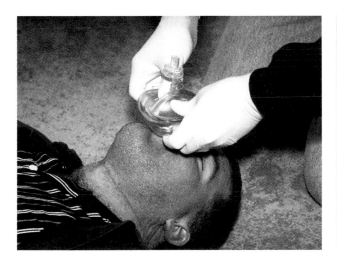

Placing a pocket mask on a patient.

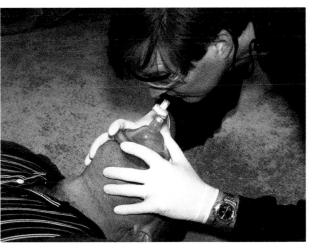

Placing the mouth over the mask's inlet port.

STOP

8. If your first breath attempt is successful, deliver one more. If your first attempt is not successful, reposition the patient's head and try again. If you are still unable to deliver air to the patient and inflate the chest, **stop**. Immediately begin FBAO removal. Continue until the patient's airway is clear or EMS arrives.

9. Once you are able to successfully deliver two breaths to the patient, perform part C of the initial assessment. Check the carotid (neck) pulse for five to ten seconds.

10. If the patient has a carotid pulse but is not breathing, you must deliver breaths to the patient once every five seconds. Continue doing this until EMS arrives. Check the carotid pulse every minute to confirm that CPR is or is not necessary.

ABDOMINAL DISTENTION

When doing rescue breathing, you must pay attention to the amount of force you use to deliver breaths. When you ventilate with too much force, air fills the lungs. Once the lungs are full, air begins to fill the stomach. Air in the stomach reduces the lungs' ability to expand and fill.

Be careful to ventilate with just enough force to expand the patient's lungs and raise the chest. Slow, deep breaths are best. If you notice the patient's abdomen getting larger, reduce the amount of force you are using.

Abdominal distention is particularly troublesome in infants and young children. Be especially careful with these patients.

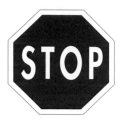 The steps for performing rescue breathing in infants and children are similar to those used for adults. One difference is that you must modify the amount of force with which you deliver breaths. Ventilating with too much force could cause abdominal distention.

The proper amount of force depends on the patient's size. An infant, for example, requires only gentle puffs of air. On the other hand, a large 7-year-old might require almost as much force as an adult.

When opening an infant's or child's airway, you must be careful to not overextend the patient's neck. Doing so can cause the airway to kink and close.

Another important consideration when ventilating infants or children is that they require more breaths per minute than adults. You must deliver 20 breaths a minute, or one every three seconds.

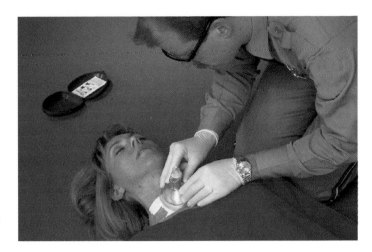

Delivering ventilations to a patient with a stoma.

VENTILATIONS THROUGH A STOMA

A person who has undergone a *laryngectomy* (removal of the vocal cords) has an opening in the neck and trachea. This is known as a *stoma*. The stoma provides a new passage for air to enter the lungs.

In very rare cases, you might need to provide ventilations to a patient with a stoma. The steps for performing this procedure are almost identical to the steps for providing ventilations through the mouth. The only difference is that the pocket mask is placed over the opening of the stoma. When ventilating a patient with a stoma, it is critical that you maintain a good seal between the mask and the skin surrounding the stoma.

While also rare, you may encounter patients who have had a partial laryngectomy. When ventilating a stoma patient who has had a partial laryngectomy, air will escape out of the patient's mouth and nose. When delivering ventilations to these patients, you must close the mouth and pinch the nose shut. This helps keep air in the airway, rather than escaping from the mouth or nose.

FOREIGN-BODY AIRWAY OBSTRUCTION: CHOKING MANAGEMENT

There are two types of FBAOs: partial and complete.

PARTIAL AIRWAY OBSTRUCTION

A partial airway obstruction allows the patient some limited air movement. It also usually stimulates a gag reflex.

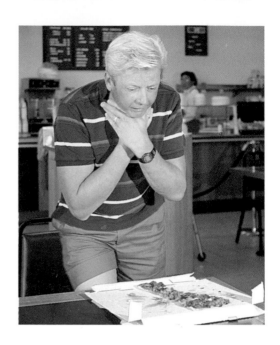

The universal sign of choking.

When a patient has a partial airway obstruction, he or she will cough, gag, and make a forceful attempt to dislodge the object. The patient may look anxious and frightened. He or she may also clutch his or her throat in the universal sign of choking.

Infants and small children will put almost anything in their mouths. That is why they choke more often than adults do. When treating a small child having difficulty breathing, look for environmental clues that may indicate an FBAO. Such clues include small objects in the carpet or reports of the child choking at the dinner table.

STEPS

PARTIAL AIRWAY OBSTRUCTION TREATMENT

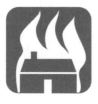

1. Ensure that the scene is safe.

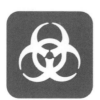

2. Take appropriate body substance isolation precautions.

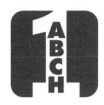

3. Perform an initial assessment. Assess the amount of air being exchanged. Determine whether the patient's gagging and coughing are effective at dislodging the object. Can the patient forcefully cough or talk? If not, immediately begin steps to expel the object.

4. If the patient is able to forcefully cough or talk, coach him or her in his or her attempts to dislodge the object.

If the partial obstruction persists:

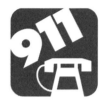

5. Activate the EMS system.

6. Monitor the patient until the object is removed or the patient is no longer able to forcefully cough or talk. In this case, the obstruction is considered complete.

7. In adult patients, do not attempt to dislodge the object with back blows or other similar techniques. Doing so can worsen the patient's condition by wasting time. It can also lodge the obstruction deeper in the airway.

COMPLETE AIRWAY OBSTRUCTION

A complete airway obstruction is a life-threatening emergency. Little or no air is able to enter or exit the airway. Occasionally, a complete airway obstruction can lead to unconsciousness and cardiac arrest.

Such an obstruction can be caused by almost any object that can be placed in the mouth. In adults, alcohol consumption is a major factor in many airway obstruction complaints.

 When an infant has a complete airway obstruction, he or she will be unable to breathe, cough forcefully, or talk. His or her skin color will turn blue, especially around the lips and fingertips.

STEPS

COMPLETE AIRWAY OBSTRUCTION TREATMENT: CONSCIOUS ADULT

1. Ensure that the scene is safe.

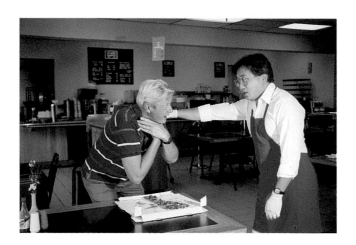

If the patient appears to be choking, ask, "Are you choking?"

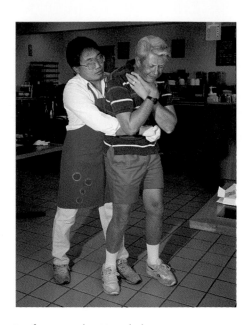

Performing the Heimlich maneuver.

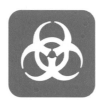

2. Take appropriate body substance isolation precautions.

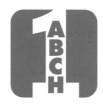

3. Perform an initial assessment. If the patient is conscious, ask, "Are you choking?"

4. If the patient is unable to respond, tell him or her that you are going to try to remove the object using the *Heimlich maneuver*.

5. Stand behind the patient. Quickly wrap your arms around his or her waist. Stabilize yourself to be able to support the patient's full weight. Place the thumb side of one fisted hand against the patient's abdomen, between the navel and the spot in the chest where the ribs join. This is called the *xiphoid process*. Grasp your fisted hand with your other hand.

6. Perform quick, upward thrusts. Push the abdomen inward and upward. Continue delivering thrusts until the object is removed or the patient becomes unconscious.

7. If the patient becomes unconscious, assist him or her to the floor. Protect his or her head and neck from injury.

8. Continue with the treatment steps for the unconscious adult with a complete airway obstruction.

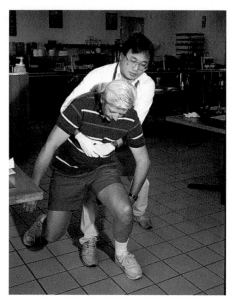

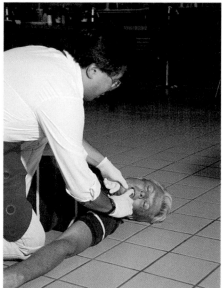

If the patient loses consciousness, assist him to the floor.

Performing the finger sweep.

STEPS

COMPLETE AIRWAY OBSTRUCTION TREATMENT: UNCONSCIOUS ADULT

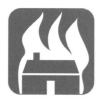

1. Ensure that the scene is safe.

2. Take appropriate body substance isolation precautions.

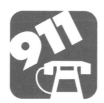

3. Activate the EMS system.

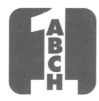

4. Perform an initial assessment.

5. If you determine that the patient has a complete airway obstruction, open his or her mouth. Do this by grasping the patient's tongue and lower jaw in one hand and lifting. Look for the object by inserting the index finger of your other hand

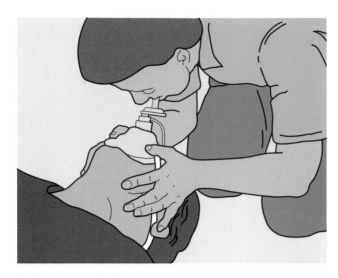

Delivering artificial ventilations.

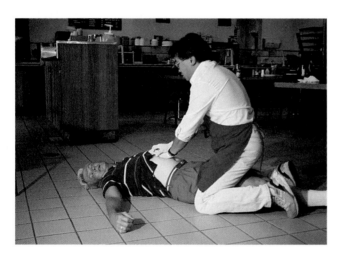

Performing abdominal thrusts.

along the inside of the patient's cheek, deep into the throat. If you find the object, use a hooking action to try to remove the object. This is called the *finger sweep*.

6. Open the patient's airway. Attempt to deliver ventilations. If your first breath attempt is not successful, reposition the patient's head, and try again.

7. If you are still unable to get air into the patient, straddle the patient with your knees outside his or her thighs. Place your hands between the navel and the xiphoid process.

8. Perform up to **five** abdominal thrusts.

9. Do a finger sweep.

DANGER

If the patient is in seizure, do not attempt to do a finger sweep.

10. Attempt rescue breathing. If you are unsuccessful, reposition the patient's head. Attempt rescue breathing again.

11. If the patient's airway remains blocked, continue steps 7 through 10 until the object is dislodged or EMS arrives.

 FBAO REMOVAL IN THE CONSCIOUS AND UNCONSCIOUS CHILD

The steps for managing FBAOs in children are similar to those for adults. One difference is that when doing the Heimlich maneuver, you must adjust the force of the thrusts you deliver depending on the size of the child. You will also typically use only one hand to reduce the amount of force applied to the abdominal cavity. Also, when treating an unconscious child, you must kneel beside, rather than straddle, the child.

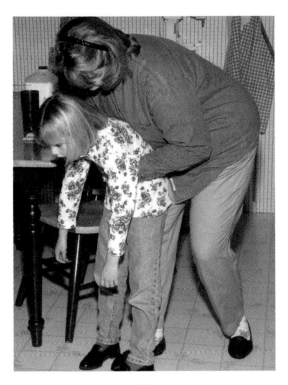

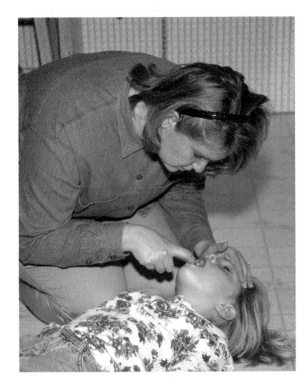

Performing abdominal thrusts in a responsive child.

When delivering FBAO treatment to an unconscious child, kneel beside—rather than straddle—the child.

STEPS

 TREATMENT OF THE CONSCIOUS INFANT WITH AN FBAO

 **1.** Ensure that the scene is safe.

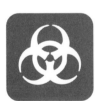 **2.** Take appropriate body substance isolation precautions.

 3. Activate the EMS system.

 4. Perform an initial assessment. Do not panic! Infants have powerful gag reflexes. Give a partial obstruction in an infant the chance to relieve itself naturally. In most cases, the object will be expelled without your help. If the obstruction is not relieved naturally or the obstruction becomes complete, begin proper FBAO techniques. Then activate the EMS system.

If a partial airway obstruction progresses to a complete airway obstruction:

5. Place the infant in the prone position. Deliver up to five back blows.

6. Flip the infant over to a supine position. Deliver up to five chest thrusts.

7. Reassess the infant's airway. Lightly pluck away any foreign objects you see in the mouth.

8. If the infant is not breathing, attempt to ventilate him or her. If your efforts are unsuccessful, reposition the infant's head. Then attempt to deliver another ventilation.

9. If you are unable to provide artificial ventilations, repeat steps 5 through 8 until the infant's airway is clear, adequate ventilations are provided, or EMS arrives.

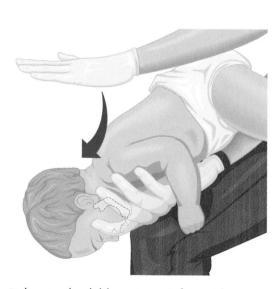

Delivering back blows to an infant with an FBAO.

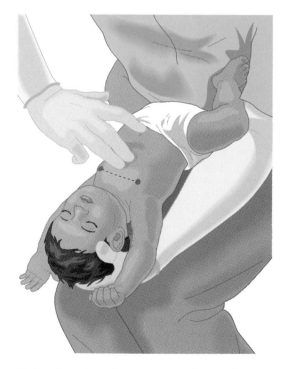

Delivering chest thrusts to an infant with an FBAO.

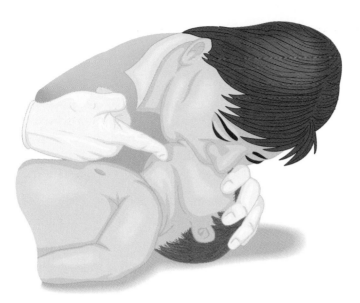

Performing artificial ventilations on an infant.

STEPS

 TREATMENT OF THE UNCONSCIOUS INFANT WITH A SUSPECTED FBAO

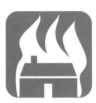 **1.** Ensure that the scene is safe.

 2. Take appropriate body substance isolation precautions.

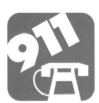 **3.** Activate the EMS system.

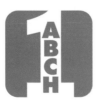 **4.** Perform an initial assessment.

If a complete airway obstruction is found:

5. Place the infant in the prone position. Deliver up to five back blows.

6. Flip the infant to a supine position. Deliver up to five chest thrusts.

7. Reassess the infant's airway. Lightly pluck away any foreign objects you see in the mouth.

8. Attempt to provide a ventilation to the infant. If your efforts are unsuccessful, reposition the patient's head. Attempt to deliver another ventilation.

9. If you are unable to provide artificial ventilations, repeat steps 5 through 8 until the airway is clear, adequate ventilations are provided, or EMS arrives.

If the patient had a significant choking event and the FBAO is relieved, encourage the infant's parents to allow him or her to be assessed by the EMS team or in an emergency department. It is critical to confirm that the object has been completely removed.

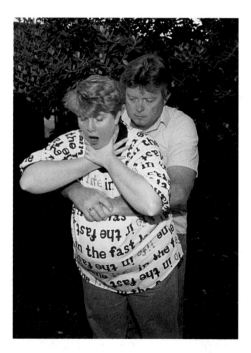

The Heimlich maneuver for pregnant or obese patients.

FBAO IN THE PREGNANT OR OBESE PERSON

The steps for treating FBAOs in pregnant or obese people are basically the same as for adults. However, when doing the Heimlich maneuver, your hand position must be higher. Your hands should be placed in the same area as when you do chest compressions in CPR (see Chapter 7).

When doing the Heimlich maneuver on a pregnant or obese patient, it is important that you do not squeeze the chest in a "bear hug." The forces caused by a bear hug are not delivered to the diaphragm, which is necessary for the Heimlich maneuver to be performed successfully. Also, a bear hug can cause severe injury to the patient's ribs. In the pregnant patient, it can also cause injury to the fetus.

CHAPTER 7

CIRCULATION AND CPR

For several years, first aid responders have been saving lives by performing cardiopulmonary resuscitation (CPR). CPR is a set of assessment techniques and hands-on procedures that attempt to restart the heart and lung functions after they have stopped. CPR can also help improve these organs' function if they are not working properly.

The CPR process includes assessing responsiveness, activating the EMS system, opening the airway, assessing breathing, performing rescue breathing (delivering artificial ventilations), checking the pulse, and performing chest compressions. You have already become proficient at performing many of these skills. Now you will learn how to perform chest compressions.

While the chances of you having to actually perform CPR are slim, if the occasion does arise, early CPR can mean the difference between life and death. That is why it is important to learn and practice your CPR skills until you are comfortable and confident performing them. Contrary to many people's opinions, CPR skills are easy to learn. If practiced often, they are also easy to recall.

Recognizing that an emergency exists and taking the proper action dramatically increase the patient's chances for a positive outcome. As a first aid responder, you are now part of the CPR chain of survival.

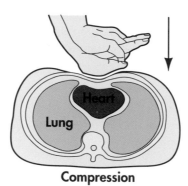 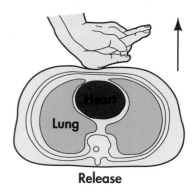

Effects of chest compressions. **Compression** **Release**

CHEST COMPRESSIONS IN ADULTS

Chest compressions are designed to circulate a patient's blood by compressing the heart between the sternum (breastbone) and the spinal column. Compressing the heart in this manner provides the patient with only about 25 percent of the blood flow normally produced by a healthy beating heart. However, that is often enough to keep the patient alive for a short time.

To perform chest compressions properly, you must first find the correct hand position. Placing your hands in any other position places the patient at risk for serious injuries. Such injuries include collapsed lungs and lacerated abdominal organs.

It is also important that you perform compressions at the proper depth. In adults, the proper depth is achieved by pressing down on the patient's chest wall approximately 1.5 to 2 inches. This depth usually equals between one-third and one-half of the patient's total chest height.

Maintaining the proper rate is also important. If you perform compressions too slowly or too quickly, the patient will not receive the correct blood flow. To top it off, you will quickly become exhausted.

Performing compressions at the proper rate allows the heart to adequately refill between compressions. The *Journal of the American Medical Association* recommends a compression rate of 80 to 100 compressions per minute in the adult patient. Compressions must therefore be performed at a rate faster than one per second. Counting techniques such as "One Mississippi, Two Mississippi, Three Mississippi" are just too slow. Instead, to achieve the proper rate of about 1.5 compressions per second, try counting as follows: "One and two and three and four and five ...."

The ratio of chest compressions to ventilations in adult CPR is 15 compressions for every two ventilations, or 15:2. Every time you complete 15 compressions and two ventilations, you have completed a cycle. In one minute of CPR, you should be able to complete four cycles.

DANGER

You must use body substance isolation precautions when delivering patient care. This is especially true during CPR events, when patients often vomit. This exposes you to body fluids. Gloves and a pocket mask should therefore be used. If a CPR event is messier than usual, you may also need to wear eye protection.

STEPS

DETERMINING THE NEED FOR CPR IN ADULTS

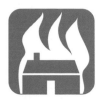

1. Ensure that the scene is safe.

2. Take appropriate body substance isolation precautions.

3. Determine the patient's level of responsiveness by using the shake and shout method.

4. If the patient does not respond, immediately activate the EMS system.

5. Perform an initial assessment. If the patient is lying on his or her stomach, gently roll him or her over. If you suspect a neck injury, have somebody help you roll the patient over. Attempt to maintain a straight line between the patient's nose and navel.

6. Open the patient's airway. If you do not suspect that the patient has spinal injuries, use the head-tilt/chin-lift maneuver. If you do suspect that the patient has spinal injuries, use the jaw-thrust maneuver.

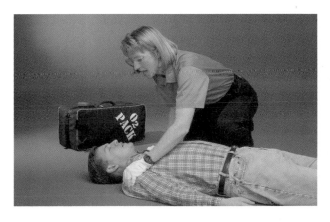

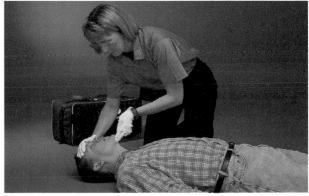

Determining the patient's level of responsiveness using the shake and shout method.

Opening the patient's airway.

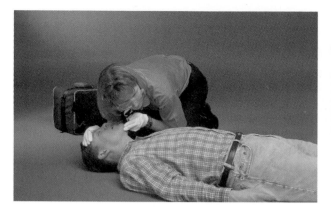

Checking to see if the patient is breathing.

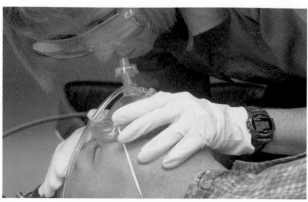

Beginning rescue breathing.

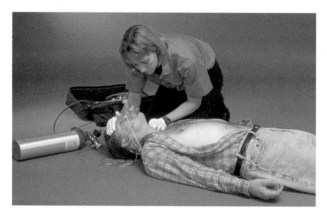

Checking to see if the patient has a pulse.

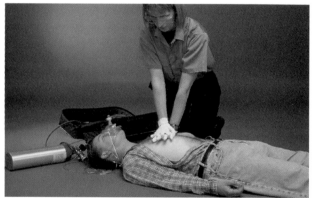

Beginning simultaneous chest compressions and rescue breathing.

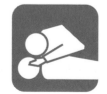

7. Check to see if the patient is breathing. If the patient is breathing and has a pulse, place him or her in the recovery position. The recovery position should not be used if you suspect a neck or back injury, however. Then continue to monitor the patient's ABCH.

8. If the patient is not breathing or is breathing less than once every six seconds, begin rescue breathing. Provide two slow breaths.

9. Check to see if the patient has a pulse.

10. If the patient does not have a pulse, begin simultaneous chest compressions and rescue breathing.

STEPS

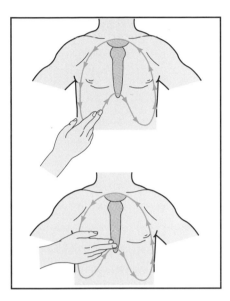

Finding the xiphoid process.

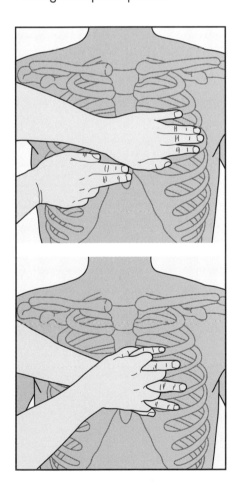

Proper hand and finger positions for performing adult CPR.

PERFORMING CPR ON ADULTS

1. To find the correct hand position, either rip away or cut off the patient's clothing. Do this as discreetly as possible. Be careful not to block the patient's airway with clothing.

2. Kneel beside the patient's chest. Run two fingers up along the rib cage. Find the junction between the two sides of the rib cage. You will feel a small, triangular-shaped bone called the xiphoid process.

3. Place your first two fingers on the xiphoid process. Then slide them approximately two finger widths up toward the patient's head. Practice finding this compression position on yourself several times.

4. Place the heel of the palm of your free hand in the center of the chest directly above your two fingers (toward the patient's head).

5. Now release your two fingers and place this hand on top of the other. Interlock your fingers. If you ever let your hand slip off the chest wall, you must start again and find the correct position.

6. Place your upper body directly over your hands. Your shoulders should be on the same vertical plane as the patient's nose and navel. Lock your arms.

7. Start doing compressions. Press down on the patient's chest wall approximately 1.5 to 2 inches. Pivot only at the hips. Try not to be alarmed if some of the patient's ribs fracture. A person who is not breathing and has no pulse is clinically dead. Breaking a few ribs while attempting to save a life is better than death. You can do it!

8. Perform a total of 15 compressions and two ventilations (one cycle).

9. Perform three more cycles, for a total of four.

10. After you have completed four cycles, or if the patient shows signs of improved consciousness such as moaning or moving, immediately stop. Check the patient's pulse for five to ten seconds.

11. If the patient has a pulse, check the status of his or her breathing. Use the head-tilt/chin-lift maneuver and the look, listen, and feel method. If the patient is not breathing, deliver ventilations. Constantly monitor the patient's pulse.

12. If the patient does not have a pulse, administer two ventilations. Then begin compressions again. Check the patient's pulse after every four cycles.

TWO-PERSON CPR TECHNIQUES

In many emergency situations, more than one first aid responder will be involved. In CPR events, more than one person can perform resuscitation skills simultaneously.

The skills used in two-person CPR are similar to those of one-person CPR. However, the compression-to-ventilation ratio is 5:1. Using this ratio, 10 cycles should be completed prior to re-assessing the patient's pulse.

When performing two-person CPR, one person performs chest compressions, while the other delivers artificial ventilations. When either responder becomes tired, he or she should ask for a change, which will take place at the end of a cycle. When changing positions, the providers should begin CPR with a breath and end with a breath.

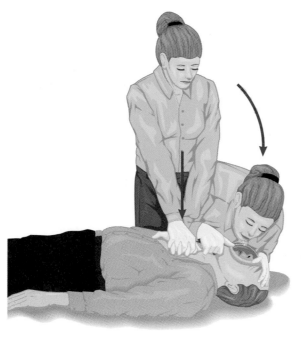

One-person CPR

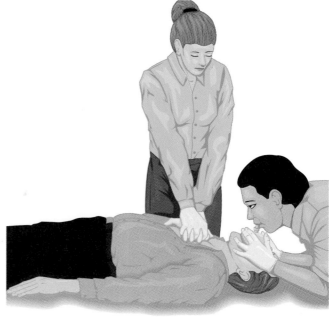

Two-person CPR

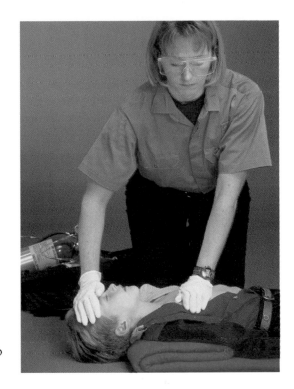

Depending on the child's size, use one or two hands to compress the chest wall.

 ## CHEST COMPRESSIONS IN CHILDREN

Performing CPR in children is similar to CPR in adults. One difference is that the depth of your compressions should be 1.0 to 1.5 inches. (Similar to adults, this depth is usually equal to between one-third and one-half of the patient's total chest height.) Another difference is that the rate at which you perform compressions is faster. You should deliver compressions at a rate of at least 100 per minute. Finally, the ratio is 5:1.

Another difference between performing chest compressions in children and adults is that with children, you will usually only need to use one hand to compress the chest wall. In this case, the other hand can be used to open the child's airway.

STEPS

 DETERMINING THE NEED FOR CPR IN CHILDREN

1. Ensure that the scene is safe.

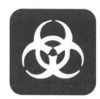

2. Take appropriate body substance isolation precautions.

3. Determine the child's level of responsiveness by using the shake and shout method.

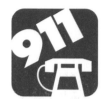

4. If the child does not respond, immediately activate the EMS system.

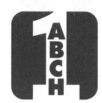

5. Perform an initial assessment. If the child is lying on his or her stomach, gently roll him or her over. If you suspect a neck injury, have somebody help you roll the child over. Attempt to maintain a straight line between the child's nose and navel.

6. If the child is breathing and has a pulse, place him or her in the recovery position. The recovery position should not be used if you suspect a neck or back injury, however. Then continue to monitor the child's ABCH.

7. If the child is not breathing or is breathing less than once every three seconds, begin rescue breathing.

8. If the child does not have a pulse, begin simultaneous chest compressions and rescue breathing.

STEPS _____

 PERFORMING CPR ON CHILDREN

1. To find the correct hand position, either rip away or cut off the child's clothing. Do this as discreetly as possible. Be careful not to block the child's airway with clothing.

2. Kneel beside the child's chest. Run two fingers up along the rib cage. Find the junction between the two sides of the rib cage. You will feel a small, triangular-shaped bone called the xiphoid process.

3. Place your first two fingers on the xiphoid process. Then slide them approximately two finger widths up toward the child's head.

4. Place the heel of the palm of your free hand in the center of the chest directly above your two fingers (toward the child's head).

5. Interlock your fingers. If you ever let your hand slip off the chest wall, you must start again and find the correct position.

6. Place your upper body directly over your hands. Your shoulders should be on the same vertical plane as the child's nose and navel. Lock your arms.

7. Press down on the child's chest wall approximately 1.0 to 1.5 inches. Pivot only at the hips.

8. Perform a total of five compressions and one ventilation (one cycle).

9. Perform 19 more cycles, for a total of 20. This should take about one minute.

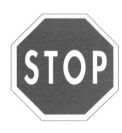

10. After you have completed 20 cycles, or if the child shows signs of improved consciousness such as moaning or moving, immediately **stop**. Check the child's pulse for five to ten seconds.

11. If the child has a pulse, check the status of his or her breathing. Use the head-tilt/chin-lift maneuver and the look, listen, and feel method. If the child is not breathing, perform rescue breathing while constantly monitoring the pulse.

12. If you do not find a pulse, administer one ventilation. Then begin compressions again. Check the child's pulse after every 20 cycles.

CHEST COMPRESSIONS IN INFANTS

Steps for performing chest compressions and CPR in the infant patient are slightly different than those for the adult or child. Simple modifications are needed to correctly perform infant CPR. One difference is that the depth of your compressions will be 0.5 to 1.0 inches. Again, this depth is usually equal to between one-third and one-half of the infant's total chest height. Another difference is that you will use only the middle and ring fingers of one hand to compress the infant's chest wall.

Similar to CPR in children, the rate at which you perform compressions in infants is at least 100 per minute. The ratio in infants is also 5:1.

STEPS

 DETERMINING THE NEED FOR CPR IN INFANTS

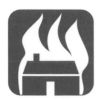

1. Ensure that the scene is safe.

2. Take appropriate body substance isolation precautions.

3. Determine the infant's level of responsiveness by gently shaking him or her. You may also shout at the infant and tickle his or her toes.

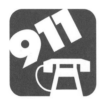

4. If the infant does not respond, immediately activate the EMS system.

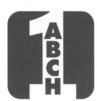

5. Perform an initial assessment.

6. If the infant is breathing and has a pulse, place him or her in the recovery position. The recovery position should not be used if you suspect a neck or back injury, however. Then continue to monitor the infant's ABCH.

7. If the infant is not breathing or is breathing less than once every three seconds, begin rescue breathing. When performing artificial ventilations on an infant, cover the infant's mouth and nose with your lips, rather than trying to pinch the nose shut. If you have a pocket mask specifically designed for infants, use it.

8. If the infant does not have a pulse, begin simultaneous chest compressions and rescue breathing.

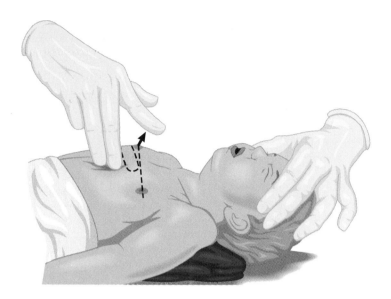

Correct hand position for delivering chest compressions to an infant.

STEPS

 PERFORMING CPR ON INFANTS

1. To find the correct hand position, either rip away or cut off the infant's clothing. Do this as discreetly as possible. Be careful not to block the infant's airway with clothing.

2. To achieve optimal compressions, the infant must be on a hard, flat surface. Place a soft towel directly underneath the infant's shoulders to place the airway in the correct position.

3. The area of compression for infants is the lower one-third of the sternum. Use an imaginary horizontal line between the infant's nipples.

4. While slightly extending the infant's head backward with one hand, place your index finger of the other hand on the patient's sternum just below the imaginary line. Now place your middle and ring fingers on the sternum, adjacent to your index finger. Raise your index finder off the infant's chest. Perform compressions with your middle and ring fingers placed approximately one finger width below the imaginary line. If you ever let your hand slip off the chest wall, you must start again and find the correct position.

5. Press down on the infant's chest wall approximately 0.5 to 1.0 inches.

6. Perform a total of five compressions and one ventilation (one cycle).

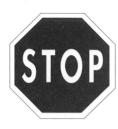

7. Perform 19 more cycles, for a total of 20.

8. After you have completed 20 cycles, or if the infant shows signs of improved consciousness such as moaning or moving, immediately **stop**. Check the infant's pulse for five to 10 seconds.

9. If the infant has a pulse, check the status of his or her breathing. Use the head-tilt/chin-lift maneuver and the look, listen, and feel method. If the infant is not breathing, perform rescue breathing. Constantly monitor the infant's pulse.

10. If you do not find a pulse, administer one ventilation. Then begin compressions again. Check the infant's pulse after every 20 cycles.

COMMON PROBLEMS DURING CPR

- Incorrect hand position.

- Incorrect compression depth.

- Failure to maintain an adequate seal around the patient's nose and mouth.

- Pivoting at the elbows or knees during compressions.

- Delivering ventilations with too much force (blowing too hard).

- Failure to maintain the proper airway position.

- Failure to activate the EMS system early enough.

- Failure to recognize either a lack of pulse or breathing.

PULSE POINTS FOR PATIENTS		
	PULSE POINT WITH RESPONSIVE PATIENT	PULSE POINT WITH UNRESPONSIVE PATIENT
Infant	Brachial	Brachial
Child	Radial or Brachial	Carotid or Femoral
Adult	Radial	Carotid or Femoral

SUMMARY OF CPR TECHNIQUES

	INFANT	CHILD	ADULT
RATIO (compressions to breaths)	5:1	5:1	15:2 (one-person CPR) 5:1 (two-person CPR)
COMPRESSION RATE	At least 100 per minute	100 per minute	80–100 per minute
COMPRESSION DEPTH	0.5 to 1.0 inch	1.0 to 1.5 inches	1.5 to 2.0 inches
BREATH RATE	20 per minute	20 per minute	10–12 per minute
BREATH LENGTH	1.0 to 1.5 seconds each	1.0 to 1.5 seconds each	1.5 to 2.0 seconds each
HAND POSITION	Two fingers on lower third of sternum	One hand on lower half of sternum	Two hands on lower half of sternum

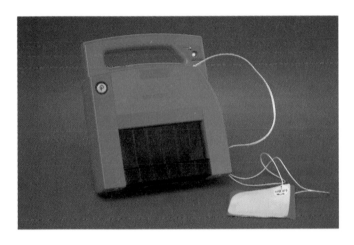

Semi-automatic AED.

AUTOMATIC EXTERNAL DEFIBRILLATORS

Research has shown that in many cases of sudden death, the use of electrical shock is beneficial in returning the heart to its normal rhythm. A device called an *automatic external defibrillator* (AED) is being used by many emergency response personnel to deliver this life-saving electrical shock.

In the near future, many first aid responders will have the opportunity to become trained in using this very valuable device.

CHAPTER 8

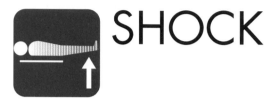 SHOCK

When the human body suffers a severe allergic reaction, loses large amounts of fluids through massive bleeding or prolonged bouts of vomiting or diarrhea, or experiences changes in the bloodstream, several body systems begin to function incorrectly. If these systems continue to function incorrectly and are left untreated, the person will go into *shock*. Once shock has progressed to its final stages, it is very difficult to reverse. In most cases, the patient dies.

As a first aid responder, it is very important that you are able to recognize the early signs and symptoms of shock. Those signs and symptoms are:

- Restlessness.
- Cool, moist skin.
- Dizziness.
- Anxiety.
- Confusion.
- Weakness.

Once you recognize that a patient is in shock, there are several first aid procedures that you can do to help slow the shock cycle and possibly save the patient's life. While there are several types of shock, at the first aid responder level, the treatment is the same regardless of the type you might encounter.

One of the best things you can do to slow the shock cycle is to help maintain the patient's normal body temperature. For example, if your patient is lying on a cold cement floor, place a blanket underneath him or her. If it's a cold day, cover the patient with another blanket. On the other hand, if it's a hot day, don't cover the patient at all.

Elderly patients and small children are much more likely to go into shock than the general population. Their bodies are weaker and are not able to correct potential problems as well as other people can. In infants and small children, you may not even see any signs or symptoms until shock has already become deadly. Always err on the side of caution. If there is any chance that a patient might be in shock, treat for shock.

STEPS

SHOCK TREATMENT

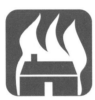

1. Ensure that the scene is safe.

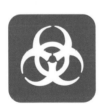

2. Take appropriate body substance isolation precautions.

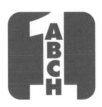

3. Perform an initial assessment.

4. Activate the EMS system.

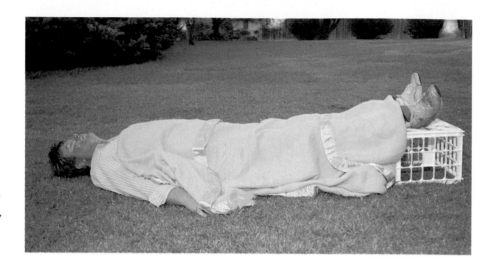

Elevate the legs of a shock patient as long as they are uninjured. In cold weather, cover the patient with a blanket.

5. Perform an ongoing assessment.

6. If the patient's legs are uninjured, elevate them approximately 12 inches. This helps shift blood away from the extremities toward the main organs of the body.

7. Help maintain the patient's normal body temperature. If it is a cold day, prevent heat loss by covering the patient with blankets or other warm items.

8. Do not give the patient any food or drink. He or she might need surgery, and the stomach should be empty.

DANGER

Patients who are in shock often vomit. This can be a problem if the patient is lying on his or her back, because saliva and vomit can pool in the airway. Be alert for airway obstructions. If necessary, carefully turn the patient onto his or her side to maintain a clear airway.

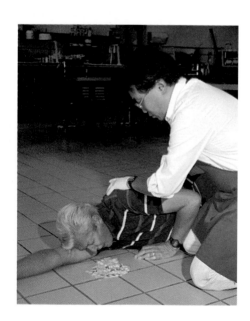

Turning the patient onto his side to help keep the airway clear.

CHAPTER 9

SOFT-TISSUE INJURIES AND BLEEDING

One of the most common types of injuries you will treat as a first aid responder is damage to soft tissue, or the skin. The emergency treatment for soft-tissue injuries is generally very basic. Despite its simplicity, proper emergency care for these wounds can have a significant impact on their overall outcome.

Soft-tissue injuries are categorized as either open (which involves a break in the skin) or closed (with no break in the skin involved). A soft-tissue injury can be an *abrasion, puncture wound, laceration, avulsion,* or *amputation.*

An abrasion occurs when the outer layers of the skin are scraped away. A puncture wound occurs when an object penetrates the skin. This can include *impaled objects.* Impaled objects can range from small pieces of metal to large fence posts. A laceration occurs when the deeper layers of the skin and muscle are cut by a sharp object. An avulsion occurs when the skin is torn away, usually leaving a flap. Finally, an amputation involves either partial or complete separation of a body part from the body.

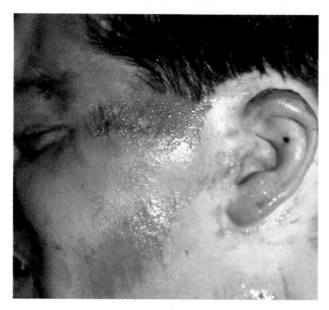

Abrasion.

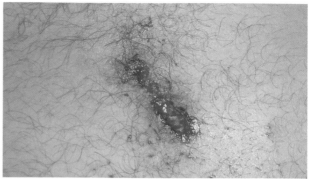

Puncture wound.

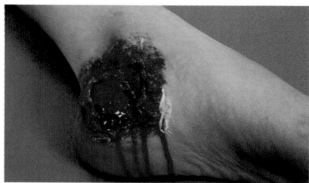

Avulsion.

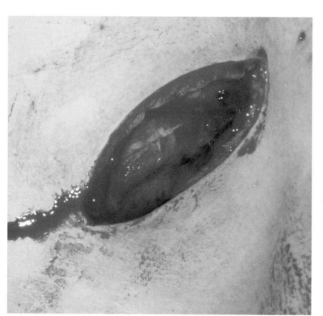

Laceration.

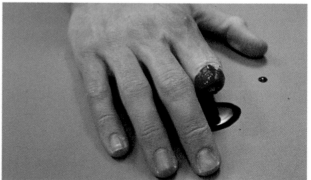

Amputation.

STEPS

TREATMENT OF GENERAL SOFT-TISSUE INJURIES WITH EXTERNAL BLEEDING

1. Ensure that the scene is safe.

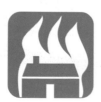

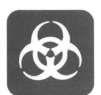

2. Take appropriate body substance isolation precautions.

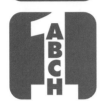

3. Perform an initial assessment.

4. If the patient is hemorrhaging, immediately apply firm, direct pressure over the wound site.

5. Perform an ongoing assessment.

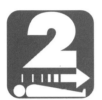

6. The treatment you deliver depends on the mechanism of injury and the type of soft-tissue injury involved. Treatment can also vary according to local protocol. Follow your instructor's advice as to what the protocol is in your area.

- In some regions of the country, treatment for lacerations, abrasions, and other cuts begins by placing fingertip pressure directly over the wound. If this doesn't control the bleeding, firm, direct pressure is then applied. The pressure applied should be equivalent to a strong handshake. This is done for a minimum of 10 minutes. In other areas of the country, treatment begins by placing a clean piece of material, such as gauze or a clean shirt, over the wound. Firm, direct pressure is then applied.

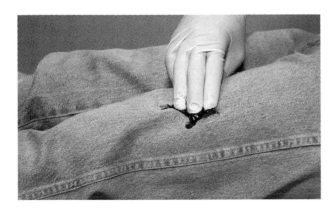

Applying direct fingertip pressure over the wound.

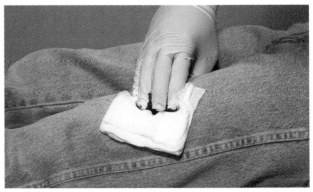

Applying direct fingertip pressure over the wound with gauze.

DANGER

Make sure that the amputated part does not come into direct contact with ice. The part also must not be packed in ice.

- If the patient has an avulsion, carefully place the flap back in the proper location. Then apply direct pressure over the wound site. Continue treatment as with any other soft-tissue injury.

- If the patient has an amputation, apply direct pressure to the stump. If possible, have another first aid responder locate the amputated part for you. Once the part is located, clean it of large debris. Then place it in a moist cloth. Place this cloth in a bag and seal it. Place the sealed bag on top of a bag of ice. Then follow the same treatment steps as with any other soft-tissue injury. Remember to always treat the patient first and then the amputated part. Be sure to transport the amputated part with the patient.

7. If a limb is involved, elevate the wounded area above the patient's heart level. If you suspect that the patient has broken bones, splint the area prior to elevation. If elevation causes an intense increase in pain, keep the extremity at the same level as the patient's heart.

8. If the bleeding continues, apply direct pressure to the patient's *pressure points*.

9. If you haven't already done so, activate the EMS system.

10. If necessary, treat the patient for shock.

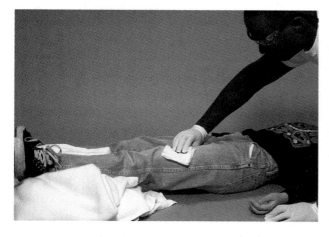

Elevating the extremity and applying direct pressure over the wound with gauze.

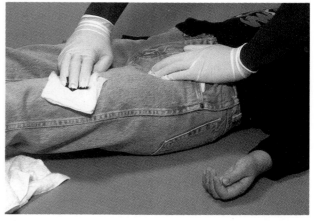

Applying direct pressure over a pressure point.

STEPS

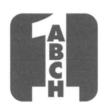

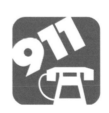

DANGER

Bleeding that is pumping or squirting from a wound, or that is severe enough to be obvious during the initial assessment, should be immediately controlled. Large wounds should be quickly covered to reduce the risk of infection.

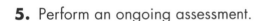

TREATMENT OF PUNCTURE WOUNDS

1. Ensure that the scene is safe.

2. Take appropriate body substance isolation precautions.

3. Perform an initial assessment.

4. If the patient is hemorrhaging, apply firm, direct pressure directly over the wound.

5. Perform an ongoing assessment.

6. The treatment you deliver will depend on the mechanism of injury and the type of puncture wound involved.

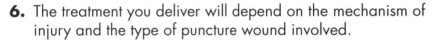

- If the patient has an impaled object, immediately activate the EMS system. In almost all cases, the next step is to stabilize the object by wrapping bulky dressings around it. One exception is if an object is impaled in the patient's cheek tissue. In this case, you may remove the object as long as it is not impaled in any other tissue. Then apply firm, direct pressure to both sides of the wound. To help control bleeding at the site of an impaled object, try to keep the patient still.

- If the patient has a sliver, attempt to remove it with a pair of tweezers. If you are unable to remove it or if the sliver is coated with toxic chemicals, it should be removed at the emergency department or nearest medical clinic.

- While rare in the workplace, you might be called on to treat human or animal bites. Bites have a high potential for infection, especially human bites. Treat all bites as soft-tissue injuries. Pay attention to bites to the patient's face or neck. These types of bites could cause bleeding into the airway. If an animal bite is suspected, secure the animal for assessment by animal control authorities.

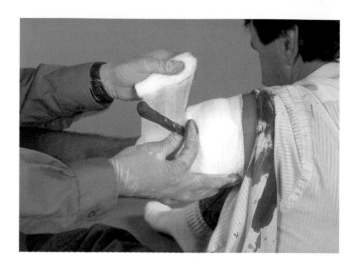

Stabilizing an impaled object.

7. If a limb is involved, elevate the wounded area above the patient's heart level. If you suspect that broken bones are involved, splint the area prior to elevation. If elevation causes an intense increase in pain, keep the extremity at the same level as the patient's heart.

8. If the bleeding continues, apply direct pressure to the patient's pressure points.

9. If you haven't already done so, activate the EMS system.

10. If necessary, treat the patient for shock.

DANGER

You must immediately control any bleeding into the airway. To drain fluids out of the airway, place the patient on his or her side. If you suspect that the patient has suffered a head or neck injury, have another person help you log-roll the patient.

NECK WOUNDS

You may occasionally encounter patients with neck wounds that are bleeding profusely. Time is critical for these patients. Major arteries and veins run through the neck. While it is important that you control bleeding, you must also focus on not allowing air to enter the bloodstream. Air bubbles can quickly kill a patient because they interrupt blood flow.

STEPS

TREATMENT OF NECK WOUNDS

1. Ensure that the scene is safe.

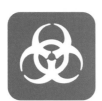

2. Take appropriate body substance isolation precautions.

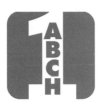

3. Perform an initial assessment.

4. If the patient has a neck wound, prevent air from entering the patient's bloodstream by placing an *occlusive* (airtight) *dressing* directly over the wound site. Commercial occlusive dressings come in a variety of sizes.

5. Place firm, direct pressure over the dressing. Be careful not to block the airway or press too hard on both arteries in the neck at the same time.

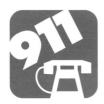

6. Activate the EMS system. Early activation is very important in patients with serious soft-tissue injuries to the neck.

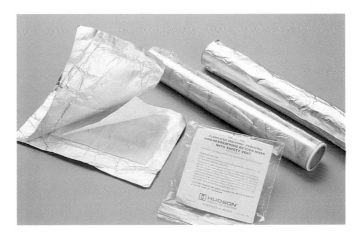

Occlusive dressings.

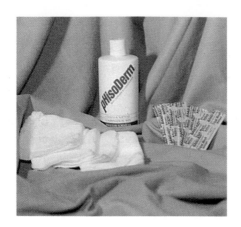

Materials for cleaning minor wounds.

STEPS

TREATMENT OF MINOR SOFT-TISSUE INJURIES

1. Ensure that the scene is safe.

2. Take appropriate body substance isolation precautions.

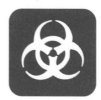

3. Clean the wound with antibacterial soap and warm water.

4. Place a nonadhesive bandage over the wound.

INTERNAL BLEEDING

Bleeding inside the body is usually caused by ruptured blood vessels, blunt trauma, decreased clotting capabilities, or serious fractures. Internal bleeding is often not recognized until shock has progressed to its late stages. That is why it is important to watch closely for the signs and symptoms of internal bleeding.

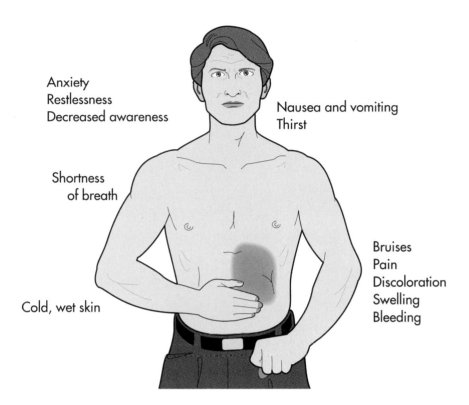

Anxiety
Restlessness
Decreased awareness

Nausea and vomiting
Thirst

Shortness
of breath

Bruises
Pain
Discoloration
Swelling
Bleeding

Cold, wet skin

Signs and symptoms of internal
bleeding.

STEPS

INTERNAL BLEEDING TREATMENT

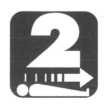

1. Ensure that the scene is safe.

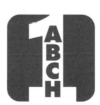

2. Take appropriate body substance isolation precautions.

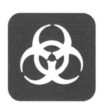

3. Perform an initial assessment.

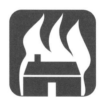

4. Perform an ongoing assessment.

5. Activate the EMS system.

6. Treat the patient for shock.

7. Administer oxygen to the patient (see Chapter 12).

8. Monitor the patient's airway. Be especially alert for vomiting.

STEPS

NOSEBLEED TREATMENT

1. Ensure that the scene is safe.

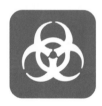

2. Take appropriate body substance isolation precautions.

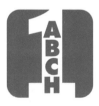

3. Perform an initial assessment.

4. Lean the patient forward to help prevent blood from being swallowed. People usually vomit after swallowing blood. If this happens, make sure the patient's airway remains clear.

5. If the nose does not look broken, pinch the patient's nostrils together. Then apply ice.

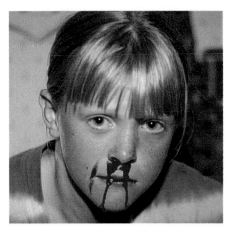

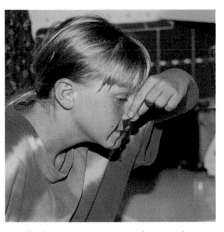

Lean the patient forward to help prevent blood from being swallowed.

Pinch the patient's nostrils together.

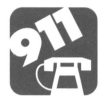

6. If necessary, activate the EMS system.

CHAPTER 10

MUSCLE AND BONE INJURIES

The human body contains more than 200 bones, 600 muscles, and several joints. As a first aid responder, your chances of treating a muscle or bone injury (*musculoskeletal injury*) are fairly high. The four major types of muscle and bone injuries are: *sprains, strains, fractures,* and *dislocations.* Fractures of the bone can be either open (which involves the bone breaking the skin) or closed (with no break in the skin involved).

Signs and symptoms of the various types of musculoskeletal injuries are very similar to each other. Most of these injuries will have signs and symptoms of pain, swelling, and occasional deformity. As a first aid responder, it is not critical that you are able to determine what type of musculoskeletal injury a patient might have. Rather, you will treat all musculoskeletal injuries, regardless of the type, by completely immobilizing (splinting) the injured area.

Immobilization is not a complicated skill. Nor is it difficult to learn. Immobilization techniques can be applied using some very basic guidelines:

- When immobilizing any area of the body, always attempt to splint the joints above and below the injured area.

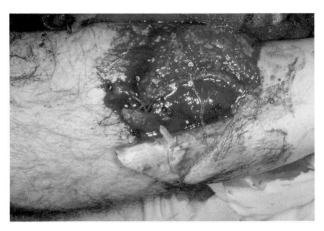

Open fracture.

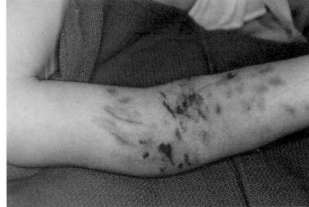

Closed fracture.

EXAMPLES OF IMPROVISED SPLINTS

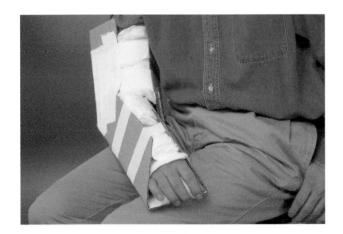

Using cardboard to splint a joint.

- Specific commercial splinting material is not necessary.

- All splints should be lightweight, sturdy, rigid, and significantly wide and long enough to support the injured area. Improvised splints work well in most situations. Look around your worksite for suitable splinting materials. Practice your splinting skills using some of these items.

- Creativity usually works best when finding a temporary splint. Do not worry about how the splint looks. Just make sure it works!

- The best (and most frequently forgotten) splint for most musculoskeletal injuries is the patient's own body.

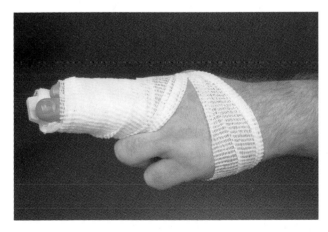

Using a tongue depressor as a splint.

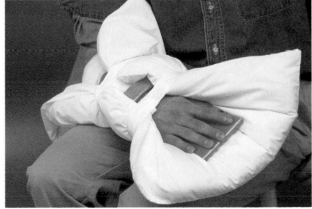

Using a pillow as a splint.

TREATMENT OF MUSCLE OR BONE INJURIES

1. Ensure that the scene is safe.

2. Take appropriate body substance isolation precautions.

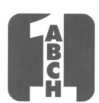

3. Perform an initial assessment.

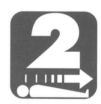

4. Perform an ongoing assessment.

5. Determine whether the muscle or bone injury is open or closed.

6. If the injury involves exposed bone ends, place clean gauze over it. Be sure not to elevate or move the injured body part. Doing so can cause additional injury.

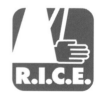

7. If the muscle or bone injury does not involve exposed bone ends, use the *RICE treatment method.*

R = Rest. This is usually accomplished by completely immobilizing the injured area. To immobilize a body part, place your splinting material next to the injured body part. Then wrap the splint with tape or gauze to keep the body part from moving.

I = Ice. Cold helps constrict blood vessels, which reduces swelling and deadens nerve endings. This in turn helps reduce pain. When you apply ice, make sure it is wrapped inside a plastic bag or some other material. Ice should not come into direct contact with the patient's skin.

C = Compression. Compression of the injured area will limit the amount of internal bleeding. To apply compression, wrap an elastic bandage around the injured area. When applying a bandage, always leave the patient's fingers and toes exposed so the advanced-level EMS providers can monitor the patient's circulation status. You may use the bandage in conjunction with an ice pack.

E = Elevation. If a limb is involved, elevate it above the patient's heart level. This will help reduce internal bleeding and swelling. This may in turn reduce the patient's pain.

8. If necessary, treat the patient for shock.

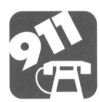

9. If necessary, activate the EMS system.

DANGER

A patient can survive without an arm or leg, but an airway that is not kept clear is deadly. Remember to prioritize the patient's problems. Your top priority is to first treat any problems that are immediately life-threatening. Muscle or bone injuries typically are not high on the list of deadly injuries.

C H A P T E R 11

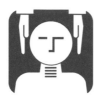 SPINAL PRECAUTIONS

One of the most potentially devastating injuries you will encounter as a first aid responder is an injury to a patient's back and spinal cord. Serious back and spinal injuries can compromise several important organ systems. Furthermore, any mishandling of the injury can cause fatal consequences for the patient. Excessive movement can cause the bones in the spine to completely sever the spinal cord. This can prevent the brain's life-sustaining signals from being delivered to the various organ systems.

It can be difficult to distinguish between a back injury that does not involve the spinal cord and one that does. You should therefore err on the side of caution when dealing with any patient who might have a back or spinal injury. You must take basic *spinal precautions* with these patients. Complete spinal immobilization will generally be accomplished by more highly trained EMS personnel.

As a first aid responder, you must be aware of situations that have a potential mechanism of injury to the back or spinal cord. Some common mechanisms of injury are:

- Motor vehicle accidents.

- Pedestrian-vehicle collisions.

- Falls.

- Blunt trauma.

- Penetrating trauma to the head, neck, or torso.

- Motorcycle accidents.

- Hangings.

- Springboard or platform-diving accidents.

- Any trauma that has left the patient unresponsive.

Patients who have suffered an injury to the back or spine may exhibit the following signs and symptoms during the initial assessment:

- Tenderness in the area of injury.

- Pain associated with movement. (Be sure to never move a potentially spine-injured patient unless his or her life is in immediate danger.)

- Pain independent of movement or palpation.

- Numbness, weakness, or tingling in the extremities.

- Paralysis or loss of sensation below the suspected level of injury.

- Paralysis or loss of sensation in the upper or lower extremities.

- Respiratory problems.

- Loss of bladder or bowel control.

Even if a patient denies having these signs and symptoms but has suffered head, neck, or back trauma, treat the patient as if a true spinal injury has occurred. Take spinal precautions, and activate the EMS system. Encourage the patient to lie still until EMS arrives.

STEPS

USING SPINAL PRECAUTIONS WHEN TREATING A PATIENT

1. Ensure that the scene is safe.

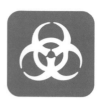

2. Take appropriate body substance isolation precautions.

3. Activate the EMS system.

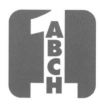

4. Perform an initial assessment. If the patient is face-down and his or her airway is blocked, use the log-roll maneuver to turn him or her over. You may also need to use the log-roll maneuver if the patient is lying on his or her back and the airway begins to fill with blood, saliva, or vomit. After rolling the patient over, clear the airway. You may have to hold the patient in this position until the airway is clear or EMS arrives.

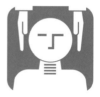

5. Take basic spinal precautions. Place your hands on either side of the patient's head to hold it still. Keep the patient's nose and navel in a straight line.

When delivering care to a patient who has been involved in a motor vehicle accident, you may be required to enter the vehicle and maintain manual stabilization of the patient's spine until EMS arrives. This is done by carefully placing your hands alongside the patient's head. Be careful not to close the patient's airway. You can use the headrest to stabilize your hands and arms. Be careful when entering and exiting the vehicle. There will likely be broken glass in the car.

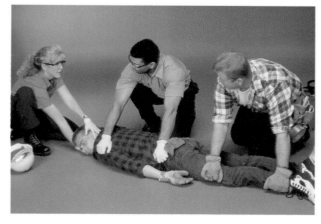

Log-rolling a prone patient.

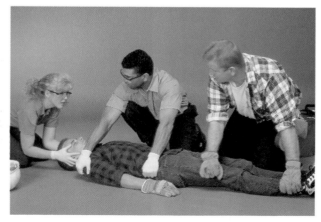

Log-rolling a supine patient.

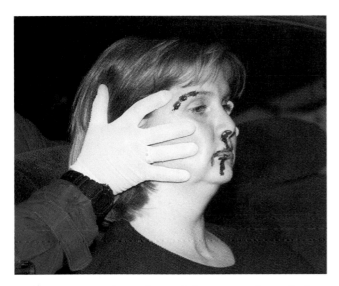

Performing manual spinal immobilization inside a vehicle.

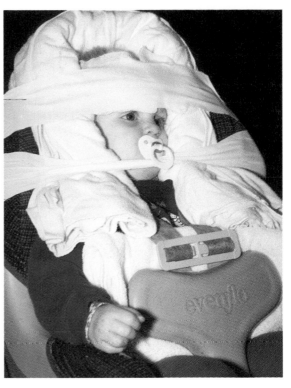

Spinal immobilization of an infant in a car seat.

6. Use the jaw-thrust maneuver to open the patient's airway. Using the jaw-thrust maneuver helps protect the patient from further injury by not moving the patient's spine.

7. If necessary, assist the patient's breathing.

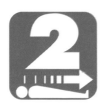

8. Perform an ongoing assessment.

9. Treat any additional injuries. Be sure not to move the patient unless the scene becomes life-threatening. If you must move the patient, use one of the emergency moves described in Chapter 2.

 As you know, infants and children are notorious for climbing up objects and falling off. Treatment for these patients is nearly identical to that for adults.

One situation you might encounter that requires slightly different spinal precautions is an infant or child involved in a motor vehicle accident who is found in a child-restraint system. Unless the child's airway is compromised, you should leave him or her in the restraint system. Gently place padding, such as rolled towels or small blankets, around the child to secure the torso and spine in place.

Carefully watch the child for any signs of airway problems. Infants and children who have head or neck injuries often vomit. Be prepared to act quickly if the child's airway becomes compromised.

CHAPTER 12

OXYGEN APPLICATION

Our bodies need an adequate supply of oxygen to function correctly. When our respiratory and circulatory systems are working properly, oxygen is inhaled into the lungs, where it attaches to red blood cells. It is then transported to every organ in the body. Several medical conditions, such as asthma, shock, and heart attacks, can adversely affect a patient's oxygen supply.

As a first aid responder, you must be able to recognize when a patient is not receiving enough oxygen. You must immediately take steps to correct the problem. This is done by delivering supplemental oxygen to the patient through a face mask or other oxygen-delivery device.

When a patient is not receiving sufficient oxygen, he or she will usually complain of *shortness of breath*, rapid breathing, anxiety, and an altered level of consciousness. Eventually, if the patient continues to receive insufficient oxygen, his or her lips, gums, ear lobes, and fingernails will turn blue.

Whenever you encounter a patient who has these signs and symptoms, you must locate an oxygen source and immediately begin administering oxygen. In most settings, oxygen delivery is accomplished through a self-contained oxygen tank and mask. If your organization does not have oxygen equipment, encourage it to get some.

As with all medical equipment, you should become familiar with the operation of your oxygen equipment **before** an emergency occurs. If possible, you should request to be formally trained in its use.

If available, oxygen should be used in the following situations:

- Chest pain.

- Difficulty breathing.

- Shock.

- Significant bleeding or soft-tissue injury.

- Burns.

- Seizures.

- Allergic reactions.

- Diabetic problems.

- Head injury.

- Abdominal pain.

There are so many other situations that warrant oxygen use that it is impossible to list them all. The bottom line is that if you are ever in doubt about whether a patient needs oxygen, administer it. Although technically considered a drug, medical oxygen will rarely hurt a patient.

Infants, young children, and the elderly can be more adversely affected by oxygen deprivation than the general population. When delivering care to these patients, you must be especially alert for breathing problems. Immediately start oxygen administration.

STEPS

OXYGEN APPLICATION

1. Ensure that the scene is safe.

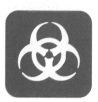

2. Take appropriate body substance isolation precautions.

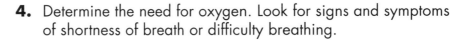

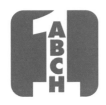

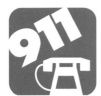

3. Perform an initial assessment.

4. Determine the need for oxygen. Look for signs and symptoms of shortness of breath or difficulty breathing.

5. Activate the EMS system.

6. Activate the oxygen delivery system. For example, turn on the main supply valve.

7. Oxygen flow typically ranges from 1 liter per minute to 15 liters per minute. As a first aid responder, you should deliver oxygen at a flow rate of between 12 liters and 15 liters per minute.

8. Place the face mask or other delivery device on the patient. Make sure the oxygen reservoir is fully inflated.

9. Monitor the patient's airway and level of consciousness.

10. Perform an ongoing assessment.

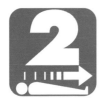

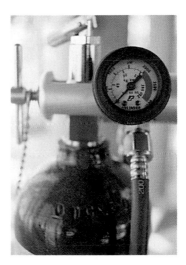

Supply valve on oxygen delivery system.

PART 2

ILLNESS AND INJURY TREATMENT

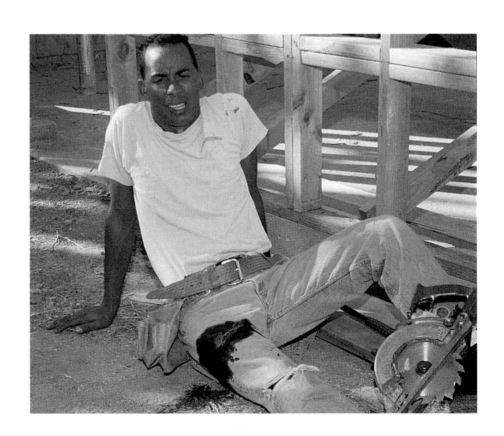

CHAPTER 13

EYE INJURIES

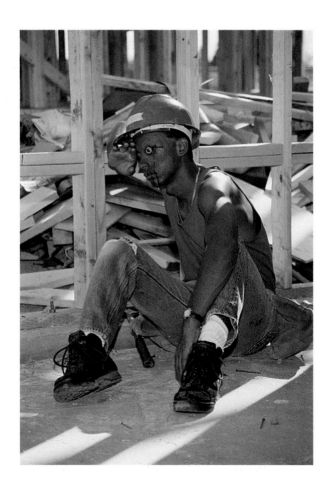

SYMBOL INDEX

Scene Safety

Body Substance Isolation

Initial Assessment

Shock

Ongoing Assessment

Soft-Tissue Care

Activation of EMS

Musculoskeletal Care

Cardiopulmonary Resuscitation

Spinal Precautions

Rescue Breathing and Artificial Ventilation

Oxygen Application

INTRODUCTION

As a first aid responder, you will likely be called on to assess and treat minor eye injuries fairly often. In many of these situations, the treatment you deliver will consist of a simple irrigation of the eye and observation of the patient. However, eye injuries can be very serious and require more advanced treatment. They can also result in a partial or total loss of vision.

It is critical that all eye-injury complaints be taken seriously. Regardless of the cause of injury, you must provide proper first aid to any patient with an eye injury.

The most common causes of eye injuries include:

- Blunt trauma, such as a hard blow to the eye area.

- Absorbed toxic chemicals, such as gasoline.

- Foreign objects, such as sawdust.

In most workplaces that have a high potential for chemical exposure to the eyes, employees are required to wear eye protection. They must also learn how to use an eye-wash station. If you have an eye-wash station in your workplace, find out how it works. Be prepared to use it.

Learning Objectives

- Recognize the different types of eye injuries.

- Demonstrate the proper first aid to be delivered in various cases of eye injuries.

EYE INJURIES: DANGER SIGNALS

If the patient has sustained any head trauma, including injury to the eye and surrounding facial bones, you must take spinal precautions before delivering any other treatment.

Never replace an eyeball that has popped out of its socket. Rather, cover the eye with a moist cloth, and wait for EMS to arrive.

If you cover an injured eye, you should always cover the uninjured eye at the same time. The patient may not like it, but it helps reduce eye movement.

Never use direct pressure on an injured eyeball.

Never remove an object impaled in the eye.

EYE INJURIES: SIGNS AND SYMPTOMS

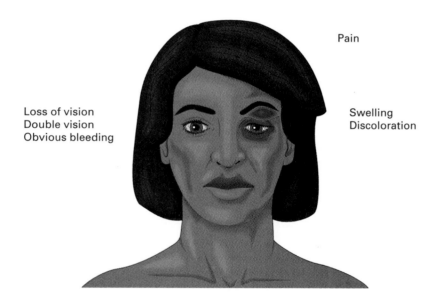

Pain

Loss of vision
Double vision
Obvious bleeding

Swelling
Discoloration

STEPS

TREATMENT OF FOREIGN-BODY EYE INJURIES AND CHEMICAL EYE INJURIES

1.    **2.** 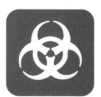   **3.**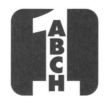

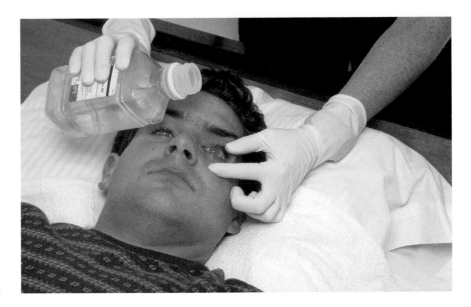

Irrigating the eye.

4. Irrigate the eye. Gently run water or another approved irrigation solution, such as saline, over the injured eye for at least 15 minutes. If it is immediately available, use warm water. Doing so causes less irritation than using cold water.

You will need another first aid responder to help you irrigate the patient's eye. One of you will irrigate the eye while the other holds the patient's eyelid open. (Having the patient try to hold his or her own eye open usually does not work very well.)

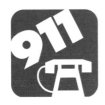

5. If the patient's pain continues after the eye is irrigated, activate the EMS system.

6. If the patient has suffered a chemical injury, try to locate and identify the chemical. Report this information to the responding EMS team.

STEPS

TREATMENT OF BLUNT TRAUMA TO THE EYE, EYE LACERATIONS, AND IMPALED OBJECTS IN THE EYE

1. 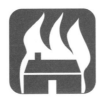   **2.** 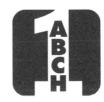   **3.**

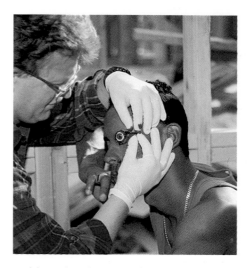

Holding the object in place.

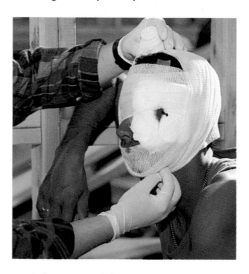

Stabilizing the object with dressings and gauze.

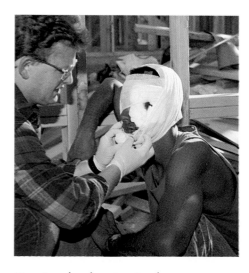

Keeping the dressing in place.

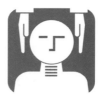

4. If the patient has suffered a blunt-trauma eye injury, take spinal precautions.

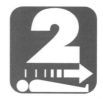

5. If the area around the eye is bleeding, apply light pressure to control the bleeding.

6. If there is an impaled object in the eye, do not attempt to remove it. You must instead stabilize the object. This is done most easily with the help of another first aid responder. One of you will firmly hold the object in place. The other will carefully place a bulky dressing around the object. The dressing is then secured in place with gauze. Once the object is secured, be extremely careful not to allow it to be bumped or hit by other objects.

Rather than attempt to stabilize the object, you may hold the object in place with two hands while waiting for EMS to arrive.

7. If the patient has suffered blunt trauma to the eye, place ice over the area surrounding the eye. This will help reduce swelling.

8. If the patient has a lacerated eye, immediately cover both eyes. Be aware that the patient will be in a great deal of pain.

9.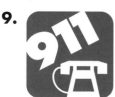

REAL-LIFE RESPONSE

You are called to assist a man who has a small piece of metal impaled in his left eye. Several of the patient's co-workers say they heard him scream and then heard a large thud. The man denies falling. He says he can remember nailing a truss together when something hit him in the eye.

The man complains of severe pain in his eye. A small amount of blood is flowing from it. The object appears to be about 2 inches long. Describe your emergency action plan.

EMERGENCY ACTION PLAN

_____

_____

_____

_____

_____

_____

_____

_____

_____

_____

_____

HEAT-RELATED EMERGENCIES

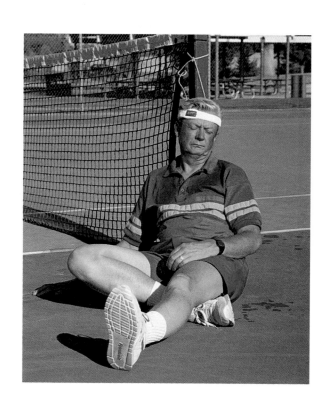

SYMBOL INDEX

 Scene Safety

 Body Substance Isolation

 Activation of EMS

 Initial Assessment

 Ongoing Assessment

 Rescue Breathing and Artificial Ventilation

 Cardiopulmonary Resuscitation

 Shock

 Soft-Tissue Care

 Musculoskeletal Care

 Spinal Precautions

Oxygen Application

INTRODUCTION

As a first aid responder, you will likely be called on to treat patients who are suffering from heat-related medical conditions. There are several types of heat-related emergencies. Some are relatively minor, but one—*heat stroke*—is life-threatening.

In hot or humid conditions, the body's ability to keep itself cool is reduced. If the person remains in the hot environment, his or her body will attempt to cool itself through sweating. Large amounts of fluids can be lost through sweating. Once enough fluids are lost without being replenished, heat-related problems can begin.

Heat cramps are another type of heat-related emergency. They are caused by the loss of important chemicals (salts) through excessive sweating. If the person remains in the hot environment and continues to sweat, he or she could progress to a more serious condition called *heat exhaustion*.

In rare cases, a patient may be unable to move from the heat and replenish the fluids he or she has lost. The patient will completely lose the ability to keep cool and will progress toward heat stroke. **Remember, this is a life-threatening emergency**. It must be treated immediately.

Learning Objectives

- Recognize the signs and symptoms of heat cramps, heat exhaustion, and heat stroke.

- Demonstrate the proper emergency care for patients suffering from heat-related emergencies.

HEAT-RELATED EMERGENCIES: DANGER SIGNALS

Very hot and dry skin is not good. It is a warning sign that the person's body has lost the ability to cool itself. It also means that heat is being retained inside the body.

Be particularly alert for heat-related problems in infants, small children, and the elderly.

 Never leave infants or small children in a parked vehicle when it is hot outside. Just a few minutes in a hot car can quickly prove fatal for small children.

The weather does not have to be extremely hot for heat-related emergencies to occur. Humidity and moderate heat can be just as bad—or worse.

Victims of heat exhaustion can appear to be fine and then rapidly progress to heat stroke.

Victims of heat emergencies commonly vomit. Be sure to maintain an open and clear airway.

HEAT-RELATED EMERGENCIES: SIGNS AND SYMPTOMS

HEAT CRAMPS

- Faintness, dizziness
- Exhaustion
- Stiff, boardlike abdomen
- Possible nausea and vomiting
- Normal mental status
- Severe muscle cramps/pain

HEAT EXHAUSTION

- Moist and clammy skin
- Pale
- Weak, dizzy, or faint
- Headache
- Nausea and vomiting

HEAT STROKE

- Life-threatening
- Dry or wet hot skin (usually red)
- Very high body temperature
- Coma or near coma

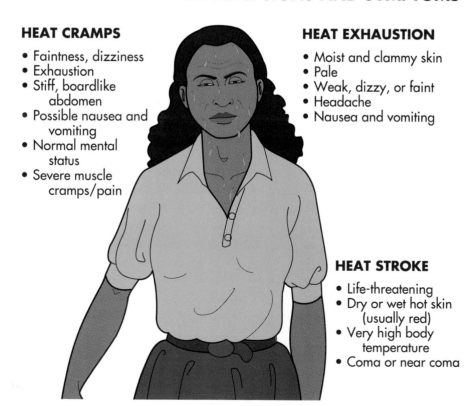

STEPS

TREATMENT OF HEAT CRAMPS AND HEAT EXHAUSTION

1.

2.

3. Move the victim to a cool area.

4.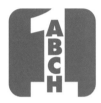

5.

6. Help cool the patient by applying damp towels or other materials to his or her skin.

7. If the patient is fully conscious, have him or her drink approximately 8 ounces (a standard-sized glass) of cool water or fruit juice every 20 minutes until signs and symptoms improve.

8.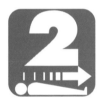

9. If the patient's signs and symptoms do not improve, activate the EMS system.

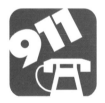

10. Instruct the patient to restrict all activity for a minimum of four to six hours.

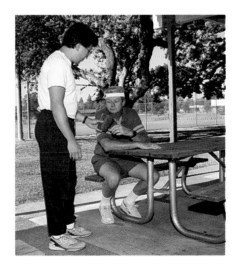

If the patient is fully conscious, have him drink 8 ounces of cool liquid.

STEPS

TREATMENT OF HEAT STROKE

1.

2.

3. Move the patient to a cool area.

4.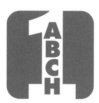

5. Monitor and treat the patient's ABCH.

6.

7. Rapidly cool the patient by removing his or her clothes. Then place damp cloths and ice packs on the groin and armpits. Fan the patient aggressively. If the patient begins to shiver, stop your cooling efforts.

8.

9.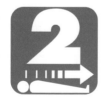

10. Continue aggressively cooling the patient until EMS arrives. Remember that heat stroke kills. Rapid and aggressive cooling action saves lives.

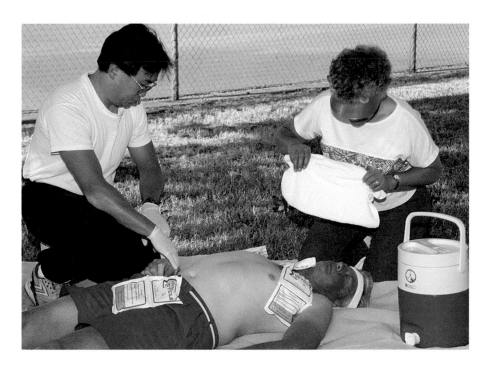

Rapidly cooling a heat stroke patient by placing damp cloths and ice packs on the armpits and groin.

REAL-LIFE RESPONSE

On a warm and humid summer afternoon, you and a friend are playing tennis. You notice an elderly man playing on a court near you. Several minutes later, you notice that the man has collapsed. You begin to assess him and note that he is weak and has very hot skin. He cannot recall what day it is. The man's partner tells you that he had cramps earlier in the day. Describe your emergency action plan.

EMERGENCY ACTION PLAN

_____

_____

_____

_____

_____

_____

_____

_____

_____

CHAPTER 15

COLD-RELATED EMERGENCIES

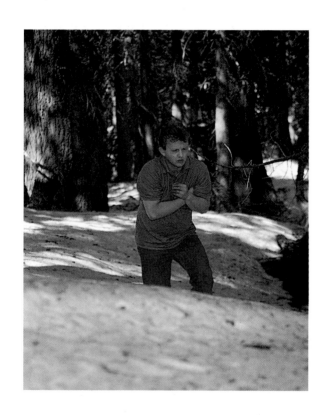

SYMBOL INDEX

Scene Safety

Body Substance
Isolation

Activation
of EMS

Initial Assessment

Ongoing
Assessment

Rescue Breathing
and Artificial Ventilation

Cardiopulmonary
Resuscitation

Shock

Soft-Tissue Care

Musculoskeletal
Care

Spinal
Precautions

Oxygen
Application

INTRODUCTION

Cold-related emergencies are a common problem in many parts of the country. As a first aid responder, you should become familiar with the various types of cold-related emergencies and their appropriate treatment.

Many people who suffer cold-related injuries are not properly prepared for rapid changes in the weather, are not prepared for extremely cold temperatures, and are unexpectedly exposed to extremely cold temperatures for long periods of time. However, similar to heat-related emergencies, cold-related emergencies can occur even if the weather is not extreme cold. For example, an elderly, partially clothed person lying on a bare concrete floor overnight can sustain cold-related injuries even if the weather outside is not extremely cold.

Patients can suffer cold-related injuries through local cooling of a body part or total body cooling. When a person is losing body heat faster than it can be produced, the person is suffering from *hypothermia*. This heat loss can be caused by many factors, such as direct or indirect contact with cool objects and wind chill.

The following factors can disrupt the body's defenses against hypothermia. While performing your ongoing assessment, you should ask the patient questions about these factors, if appropriate:

- Weather severity.

- Age. Infants and the elderly are at higher risk of hypothermia than the general population.

- Pre-existing medical conditions, such as cardiac problems or diabetes.

- Alcohol or drug consumption.

- Clothing.

Learning Objectives

■ Demonstrate the ability to recognize the signs and symptoms of cold-related emergencies.

■ Demonstrate the proper assessment and treatment of patients suffering from local or general body cooling.

COLD-RELATED EMERGENCIES: DANGER SIGNALS

If a person has been reported missing in an excessively cold area, such as the mountains, do not attempt to participate in search and rescue efforts unless you are specially trained to do so.

If there is any chance that frozen body parts will freeze again before professional treatment can be delivered, do not attempt to warm them.

Be aware of your own limits. When working in a cold environment, watch for signs of cold-related injury in yourself and your fellow first aid responders. Always wear appropriate clothing.

Handle all hypothermia patients very gently. Even though people suffering from hypothermia may not feel pain in the area that is frozen, it is important to handle them gently to avoid causing additional injury.

STAGES OF HYPOTHERMIA

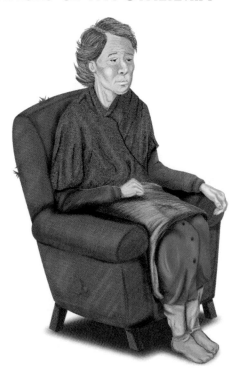

1. Shivering

2. Feeling of numbness

3. Slow breathing

4. Slow pulse

5. Slurred speech

6. Decreasing levels of consciousness

7. Hard, cold, painless body parts

8. Death

TREATMENT OF COLD-RELATED EMERGENCIES

1. Make sure you are adequately protected from the elements by wearing appropriate clothing.

2.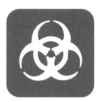

3.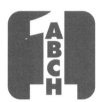

4. If possible, move the patient to a warm area.

5.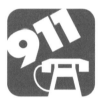

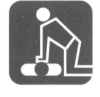

6. If necessary, perform CPR.

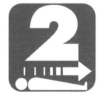

7. Keep the patient still, remove all wet clothing, and cover him or her with blankets. Assess the patient for frostbite.

8. If necessary, treat the patient for shock.

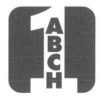

9. Maintain the patient's airway. Repeat the initial assessment as necessary. Monitor and treat the patient's ABCH.

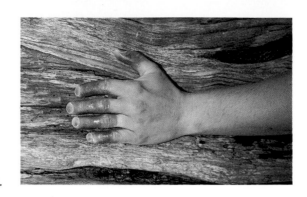

Frostbitten fingers.

REAL-LIFE RESPONSE

While driving in the mountains on a cold afternoon, you stop along the road to have lunch in the car. While eating, you see a young man staggering through the trees. You begin to deliver care to the man and determine that he has been out in the snow for several hours after his car broke down. He is cold to the touch. He is blue around the lips, ears, and hands. He is slightly confused. Describe your emergency action plan.

EMERGENCY ACTION PLAN

_____

_____

_____

_____

_____

_____

_____

_____

_____

_____

_____

CHAPTER 16

BURNS

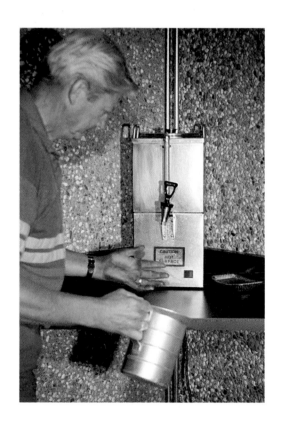

SYMBOL INDEX

 Scene Safety

 Body Substance Isolation

 Activation of EMS

 Initial Assessment

 Ongoing Assessment

 Rescue Breathing and Artificial Ventilation

 Cardiopulmonary Resuscitation

 Shock

 Soft-Tissue Care

 Musculoskeletal Care

 Spinal Precautions

 Oxygen Application

INTRODUCTION

Burns are a type of soft-tissue injury. If severe enough, they can be one of the most devastating injuries you will treat as a first aid responder. The major types of burns are:

- Thermal (flame, air, steam).
- Chemical (dry and liquid).
- Electrical.
- Radiation.

Burns are classified as *first-degree*, *second-degree*, and *third-degree* according to their severity.

Learning Objectives

- Identify the major types of burns.
- Identify the signs and symptoms associated with first-, second-, and third-degree burns.
- Demonstrate proper first aid for first-, second-, and third-degree burns.
- Demonstrate proper first aid for burns caused by dry or liquid chemicals.

BURNS: DANGER SIGNALS

In all burn emergencies, you must be absolutely sure to assess the safety of the scene. Never enter a scene unless you are absolutely sure of your safety. Fires release many odorless, colorless toxic gases, which can quickly kill.

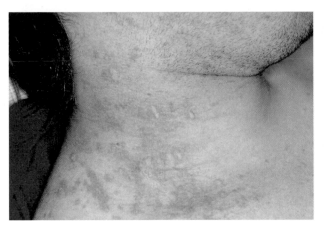

First-degree burn.

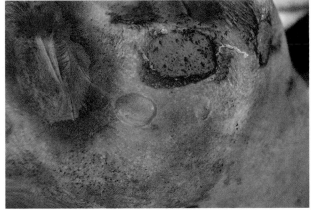

Third-degree burn.

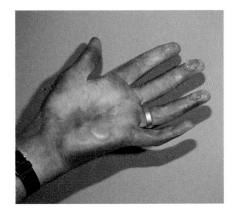

Second-degree burn.

Burn injuries can expose you to various body fluids. Be sure to take appropriate body substance isolation precautions.

When treating a victim of a chemical burn, brush off all dry chemicals prior to irrigating the burn.

If a large area of the patient's skin is burned, even if it is the less critical first-degree or second-degree type, you must activate the EMS system immediately.

BURN SEVERITY: SIGNS AND SYMPTOMS

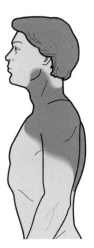

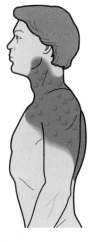

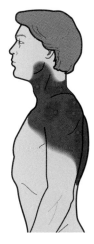

FIRST-DEGREE
Pain
Red skin
Swelling

SECOND-DEGREE
Pain
Blistering
White or red skin
Body fluids leaking from
    the burn site

THIRD-DEGREE
Minimal pain at the burn
    site
Multicolored skin (black,
    white, gray, and red)
Severe body fluid loss

STEPS

TREATMENT OF FIRST-DEGREE THERMAL, ELECTRICAL, AND RADIATION BURNS

1.

2.

3.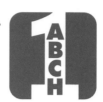

4.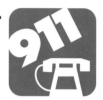

5.

6. If an extremity is burned, place the injured area in cool water for 20 minutes. If the injured area is not an extremity, cover the burn with a cool cloth. Replace the cloth with a new one every few minutes to help cool the area and reduce swelling.

7. Once the burned area is cool, cover it with a dry bandage.

STEPS

TREATMENT OF SECOND-DEGREE THERMAL, ELECTRICAL, AND RADIATION BURNS

1.

2.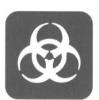

3.

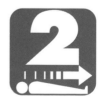

4. Remove all jewelry. This will help prevent constriction as the burn area swells.

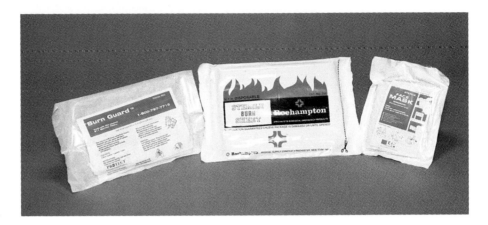

Commercial burn sheets.

5.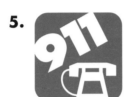

6. Cover the injured area with a dry, nonstick cloth or sheet. If available, you should use commercial burn sheets.

7.

8. If necessary, treat the patient for shock.

STEPS

TREATMENT OF THIRD-DEGREE THERMAL, ELECTRICAL, AND RADIATION BURNS

1.   **2.**   **3.**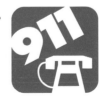

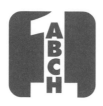

4. If necessary, stop the burning process by extinguishing any clothes that are on fire. You may also need to remove any clothing that is still hot, such as belt buckles.

5.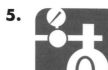

6. Remove any jewelry.

7. Cover the injured area with a dry, nonstick cloth or sheet. If available, you should use commercial burn sheets.

8. If necessary, treat the patient for shock.

9. Re-evaluate the patient. Maintain and treat the patient's ABCH.

STEPS

TREATMENT OF FIRST-, SECOND-, AND THIRD-DEGREE CHEMICAL BURNS

1.   **2.** 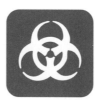   **3.**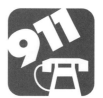

4. Determine if the chemical is liquid or dry. If the chemical is dry, rapidly brush it off. Make sure your hands and face are protected as you brush off the chemical.

5.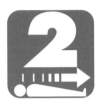

6. Rapidly irrigate the burned area with water.

7.

8. Continue irrigating the burned area.

9.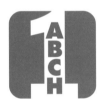

10. Attempt to identify the chemical by checking container labels or, if applicable, material safety data sheets.

11. Re-evaluate the patient. Maintain and treat the patient's ABCH.

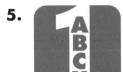

Burns in infants and children can be extremely dangerous—even those that do not look severe. Burns in infants and children damage more surface area in relation to the patient's total body size than in adults. This in turn causes greater fluid and heat loss and greater risk of infection.

When treating any infant or child with a burn injury, make sure to treat the burn appropriately. Keep the patient's body temperature as normal as possible. One way to help maintain the patient's normal body temperature is to use commercial burn sheets. They help maintain the patient's body temperature while reducing the chance of infection.

REAL-LIFE RESPONSE

As the owner of an auto repair company, you are frequently called on to replace car batteries. While helping a fellow worker replace a newly charged battery, the battery suddenly explodes in your employee's face. His entire face and chest are burned and quickly become covered with small blisters. The burns appear to be second-degree. The patient complains of having slight difficulty breathing and burning in his eyes. Describe your emergency action plan.

EMERGENCY ACTION PLAN

_____

_____

_____

_____

_____

_____

_____

_____

_____

_____

C H A P T E R 17

BREATHING EMERGENCIES

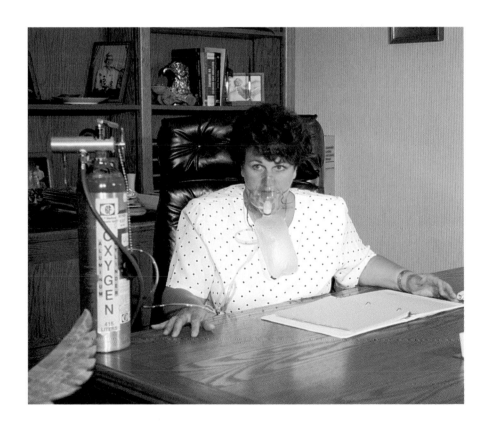

SYMBOL INDEX

Scene Safety

Body Substance Isolation

Activation of EMS

Initial Assessment

Ongoing Assessment

Rescue Breathing and Artificial Ventilation

Cardiopulmonary Resuscitation

Shock

Soft-Tissue Care

Musculoskeletal Care

Spinal Precautions

Oxygen Application

INTRODUCTION

Breathing emergencies are one of the most common problems you will encounter as a first aid responder. While some of these problems are fairly minor, others can become life-threatening if they are not cared for quickly and appropriately.

It is important that you are able to determine when a patient is experiencing breathing emergencies. More importantly, when delivering care to a patient with breathing problems, you must be able to recognize when those problems are worsening. Early recognition of breathing emergencies, appropriate basic first aid, and activation of the EMS system can have a major impact on the patient's outcome.

Many patients who are in the midst of a breathing emergency will deny that they are having a problem and will refuse to allow you to care for them. If you encounter this type of situation, activate the EMS system, and let the advanced-level EMS personnel evaluate the patient.

There are numerous causes of breathing emergencies. The most common causes include:

- Asthma, croup, and *bronchiolitis*.

- Allergies.

- Heart problems.

- Inhalation injuries, such as from gases.

- Smoking.

- Lung diseases.

- *Hyperventilation*.

Learning Objectives

- Recognize the various signs and symptoms of breathing emergencies.
- Describe and demonstrate the proper emergency care for the patient complaining of breathing emergencies.

BREATHING EMERGENCIES: DANGER SIGNALS

Breathing emergencies can progress from minor discomfort to life-threatening shortness of breath in a matter of minutes. Be sure to carefully monitor the patient's breathing rate and effort. These signs can offer early clues as to when a breathing emergency is worsening.

BREATHING EMERGENCIES: SIGNS AND SYMPTOMS

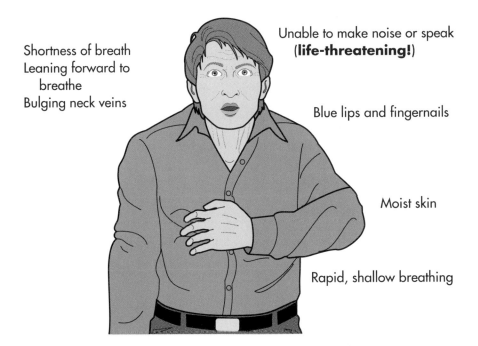

Shortness of breath
Leaning forward to
   breathe
Bulging neck veins

Unable to make noise or speak
(**life-threatening!**)

Blue lips and fingernails

Moist skin

Rapid, shallow breathing

STEPS

TREATMENT OF BREATHING EMERGENCIES

1.

2.

3.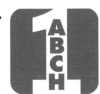

4. If the patient is able to take his or her own prescribed respiratory medication, encourage him or her to do it.

5.

6.

Like adults, infants and children can experience breathing emergencies. You must take special care when performing an initial assessment on these patients. Infants and children are generally able to tolerate respiratory distress for some time without showing any obvious signs. However, they will suddenly run out of energy, and their condition will deteriorate rapidly. Carefully determine the rate and quality of the infant's or child's breathing, and watch for changes in rate, quality, and effort. Pay particular attention to the infant or child who looks too tired to breathe.

BREATHING EMERGENCIES IN INFANTS AND CHILDREN: SIGNS AND SYMPTOMS

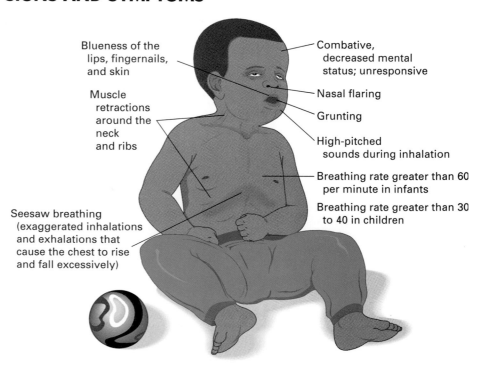

Blueness of the lips, fingernails, and skin

Muscle retractions around the neck and ribs

Seesaw breathing (exaggerated inhalations and exhalations that cause the chest to rise and fall excessively)

Combative, decreased mental status; unresponsive

Nasal flaring

Grunting

High-pitched sounds during inhalation

Breathing rate greater than 60 per minute in infants

Breathing rate greater than 30 to 40 in children

In some cases, it may be very difficult to see signs of breathing emergencies in infants and children. A subtle yet telling sign is unnatural restlessness or agitation. If a child cannot breathe properly, his or her level of consciousness will eventually change. The child may then act restless or irritable. This can be a first sign that it is becoming difficult to breathe.

Never underestimate a child's complaint of having difficulty breathing. When children experience breathing emergencies and get to the point that their breathing is slowing, they are exhausted and are about to stop breathing altogether.

REAL-LIFE RESPONSE

You are in your office when a fellow employee comes in and tells you that your manager is having problems breathing. When you question your manager, she tells you that she has been having trouble breathing for about an hour. She also tells you that she has asthma. She admits that she is under a lot of stress and says she does not want to go to the hospital. She has a prescription breathing medication in her purse but failed to take her daily dose before work. Describe your emergency action plan.

EMERGENCY ACTION PLAN

_____

_____

_____

_____

_____

_____

_____

_____

_____

_____

_____

CHAPTER 18

CARDIAC EMERGENCIES: CHEST PAIN AND HEART ATTACKS

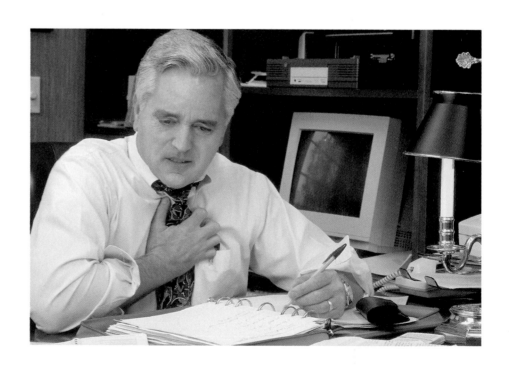

SYMBOL INDEX

Scene Safety

Body Substance Isolation

Activation of EMS

Initial Assessment

Ongoing Assessment

Rescue Breathing and Artificial Ventilation

Cardiopulmonary Resuscitation

Shock

Soft-Tissue Care

Musculoskeletal Care

Spinal Precautions

Oxygen Application

INTRODUCTION

Cardiac emergencies are one of the most complicated medical complaints you will manage as a first aid responder. They are also one of the most time-sensitive. In fact, time is the No. 1 enemy of patients suffering from cardiac emergencies.

Most people who experience a cardiac emergency will wait several hours before requesting help. If these people are having a heart attack, their heart muscle will continue to die while they wait. Unfortunately, this hesitation or unwillingness to seek emergency medical care often proves deadly.

As a first aid responder, you should help educate the public about the importance of activating the EMS system immediately for all patients who are complaining of chest pain or cardiac emergencies—regardless of how insignificant their signs and symptoms might seem. The heart is the pump of life. Without an effective pump, death is inevitable.

You may also want to discuss with your local EMS agency the possibility of integrating the automatic external defibrillator (AED) into your first aid response to cardiac emergencies. This new technology holds great promise for increased survival rates from sudden cardiac death.

Learning Objectives

- Recognize the signs and symptoms of chest pain and heart attacks.

- Understand and perform emergency treatment for patients suffering chest pain and possible heart attacks.

CARDIAC EMERGENCIES: DANGER SIGNALS

Anticipate denial. For various reasons, many patients will deny having chest pain and refuse medical care. Don't be timid. You may need to give the patient some friendly yet strong advice. When responding to any cardiac patient who refuses your care, activate the EMS system early. EMS responders are very good at convincing people of the need for medical care.

CARDIAC EMERGENCIES: SIGNS AND SYMPTOMS

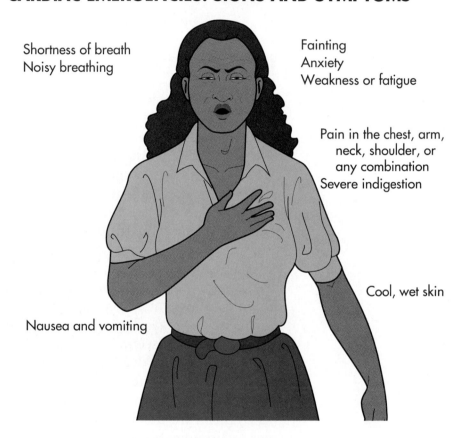

Shortness of breath
Noisy breathing

Fainting
Anxiety
Weakness or fatigue

Pain in the chest, arm, neck, shoulder, or any combination
Severe indigestion

Cool, wet skin

Nausea and vomiting

STEPS

TREATMENT OF CARDIAC EMERGENCIES

1.

2.

3.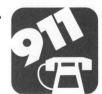

4.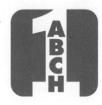

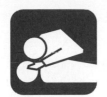

5. If necessary, deliver artificial ventilations.

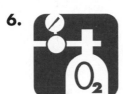

6.

7. If necessary, perform CPR.

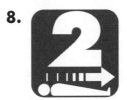

8.

REAL-LIFE RESPONSE

While eating at a restaurant, you notice an elderly man rubbing the center of his chest and complaining to the staff about chest pain. As you question the man, he tells you that he had a mild heart attack five years ago. The patient complains of chest pain that moves up his left arm. He is cool, pale, and sweaty. Just as you are about to call 9-1-1, the man slumps to the floor and loses consciousness. Describe your emergency action plan.

EMERGENCY ACTION PLAN

_____

_____

_____

_____

_____

_____

_____

_____

_____

CHAPTER 19

CHEST AND HEAD INJURIES

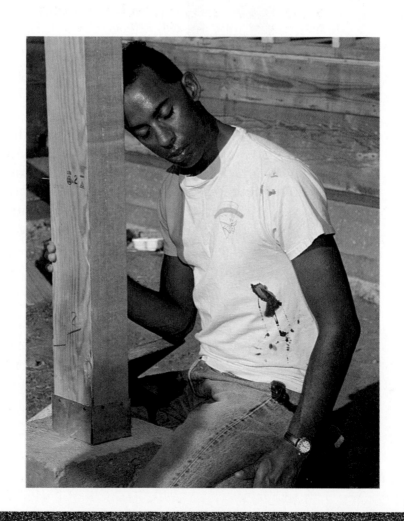

SYMBOL INDEX

 Scene Safety

 Body Substance Isolation

 Activation of EMS

 Initial Assessment

 Ongoing Assessment

 Rescue Breathing and Artificial Ventilation

 Cardiopulmonary Resuscitation

 Shock

 Soft-Tissue Care

 Musculoskeletal Care

 Spinal Precautions

 Oxygen Application

INTRODUCTION

Injuries to the chest or head can cause massive internal and external bleeding. These injuries can also be associated with underlying damage to the face, eyes, brain, airway, spine, lungs, heart, and ribs. When treating any patient with significant chest or head injuries, you must do your best to keep the patient still. This will help reduce the risk of additional injury. If you must move the patient for any reason, such as to help clear an obstructed airway, be sure to use spinal precautions.

CHEST INJURIES

Due to the size and location of the chest, patients involved in traumatic accidents often suffer chest injuries. These patients can also have serious injuries to the organs in the chest cavity. The lungs, diaphragm, heart, and major blood vessels can be severely damaged in cases of chest trauma. Because of the potential of injury to these organs, you must pay close attention to the patient's breathing effort during your initial assessment.

During your ongoing assessment, you must carefully assess the patient's chest wall for injuries. One common type of injury to the chest wall is fractured ribs. In this type of situation, the patient may have a simple single-rib fracture or multiple ribs fractured in multiple locations. This latter injury is called *flail chest*.

The injury may also have been caused by a penetrating object, such as a knife or bullet. When the chest wall is penetrated in this manner, air is sucked through the wound site into the chest. This can cause the lung to collapse. As air becomes trapped inside the chest cavity, the patient's ability to breathe is severely hindered. This type of injury is known as a *sucking chest wound*. **It is extremely life-threatening**.

Chest Injuries: Learning Objectives

- Identify the signs and symptoms of chest injuries.
- Recognize the different types of chest injuries.
- Describe the proper emergency care for chest injuries.

CHEST INJURIES: DANGER SIGNALS

Chest injuries are always serious because of their ability to hinder breathing. In all cases of chest injury, you must immediately activate the EMS system.

Many chest injuries show little or no signs of external injury. Always err on the side of caution and assume the worst. Internal chest injuries can quickly kill your patient.

CHEST INJURIES: SIGNS AND SYMPTOMS

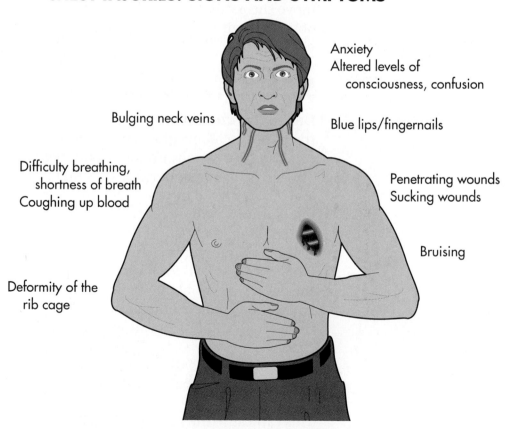

Anxiety
Altered levels of
  consciousness, confusion

Blue lips/fingernails

Bulging neck veins

Difficulty breathing,
  shortness of breath
Coughing up blood

Penetrating wounds
Sucking wounds

Bruising

Deformity of the
rib cage

STEPS

TREATMENT OF RIB FRACTURES, FLAIL CHEST, PENETRATING WOUNDS, AND SUCKING CHEST WOUNDS

1.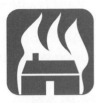

2.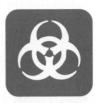

3.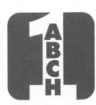

4.

5.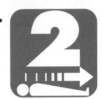

6.

7.

8. If the patient has a penetrating chest wound or a sucking chest wound, immediately place your gloved hand over the wound. Then place a piece of aluminum foil or other airtight dressing over the wound. Make sure air is not entering the wound site.

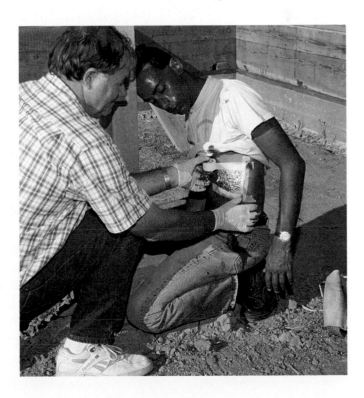

Placing an occlusive dressing over a chest wound.

REAL-LIFE RESPONSE

While delivering lumber to a large construction site, you hear someone screaming for help. You look for the person and find a man lying on the concrete. He is moaning in pain. He appears to be about 25 years old. The patient says he fell from a ladder from a height of about 12 feet. You notice that the patient is having difficulty breathing. Describe your emergency action plan.

EMERGENCY ACTION PLAN

_____

_____

_____

_____

_____

_____

_____

_____

_____

_____

_____

_____

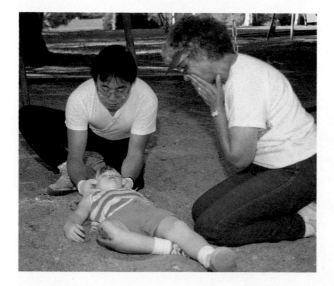

HEAD INJURIES

In patients with head injuries, bleeding under the skull can begin immediately after the injury is sustained. It can also be delayed for hours.

One of the best ways to determine if internal bleeding is occurring is to watch for changes in the patient's level of consciousness. Remember, a patient can have massive internal bleeding without having any external bleeding wounds to the head. If the mechanism of injury is significant, you must assume that the patient has sustained an internal head injury until proven otherwise. Take spinal precautions in all cases of significant head trauma.

If the patient has both head injuries and soft-tissue injuries to the face or throat, first take all necessary precautions to protect the airway and spine. Then treat the soft-tissue injuries. (Review Chapter 9 for special steps required for some throat injuries.)

As mentioned in Chapter 11, infants and children have a knack for falling off things. Minor bumps and bruises—including on the head—are a part of growing up. In many cases, these injuries consist of a minor bump that disappears after a few hours with the help of a little ice to reduce the swelling.

While there is no simple rule for assessing the severity of these bumps and bruises, one rule can help you decide when to treat an infant or child's head injury as serious. If an infant or child is knocked unconscious for any length of time, if the child vomits after the injury, or if you simply do not feel comfortable with the injury, activate the EMS system immediately.

Head Injuries: Learning Objectives

- Recognize the signs and symptoms of a head injury.

- Demonstrate the proper emergency treatment for a head injury.

- Understand the importance of spinal precautions and airway management in all patients with head injuries.

HEAD INJURIES: DANGER SIGNALS

All patients with significant head injuries should be treated as if they have an accompanying spinal injury. Spinal precautions should be taken with these patients.

Many patients with head injuries vomit. If the patient does vomit, maintain a clear airway by turning the patient onto his or her side. Be sure to use spinal precautions as you turn the patient.

Some patients who have a head injury will at first appear fine and then rapidly lose consciousness.

Patients with severe facial injuries usually have airway problems. Be sure to keep the airway clear.

HEAD INJURIES: SIGNS AND SYMPTOMS

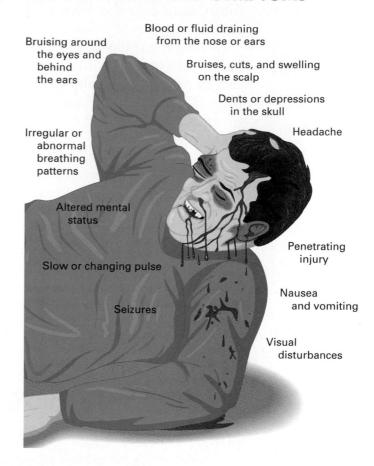

Bruising around the eyes and behind the ears

Blood or fluid draining from the nose or ears

Bruises, cuts, and swelling on the scalp

Dents or depressions in the skull

Headache

Irregular or abnormal breathing patterns

Altered mental status

Slow or changing pulse

Seizures

Penetrating injury

Nausea and vomiting

Visual disturbances

STEPS

TREATMENT OF HEAD INJURIES

1.

2.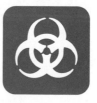

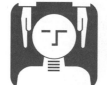 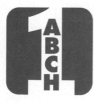

3. Pay particular attention to the patient's airway. Make sure it remains clear of blood, vomit, and saliva.

4.

5.

6. Do not use firm, direct pressure on the wound. Make sure to not press too hard on the skull.

7.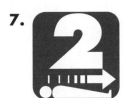

8. If necessary, treat the patient for shock.

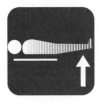

REAL-LIFE RESPONSE

While you are working in the kitchen of a busy restaurant, a fellow employee slips on some cooking oil and strikes his head. As you question the patient, you find that he momentarily lost consciousness. He complains of head pain and nausea. You notice a small cut on the back of his head. Describe your emergency action plan.

EMERGENCY ACTION PLAN

_____

_____

_____

_____

_____

_____

_____

_____

_____

CHAPTER 20

ABDOMINAL EMERGENCIES

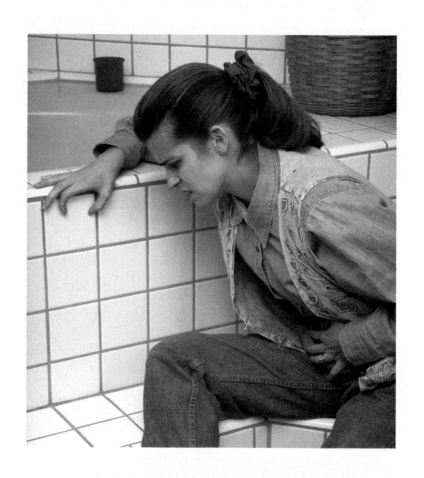

Scene Safety

Body Substance Isolation

Activation of EMS

Initial Assessment

Ongoing Assessment

Rescue Breathing and Artificial Ventilation

Cardiopulmonary Resuscitation

Shock

Soft-Tissue Care

Musculoskeletal Care

Spinal Precautions

Oxygen Application

INTRODUCTION

Abdominal emergencies can be a challenge to even the most experienced first aid responder. These types of emergencies, which include abdominal injuries and complaints of abdominal pain, are often difficult to assess and manage. Patients suffering from abdominal emergencies will complain of generalized pain and discomfort. They are often unable to pinpoint the exact location of their pain.

Abdominal emergencies can be caused by blunt trauma, such as a direct blow; penetrating trauma, such as a stabbing; diseases, such as cancer; blockages, such as an impacted bowel; and other medical conditions, such as a tubal pregnancy. Despite their potential for being serious, abdominal emergencies are often seen as minor by many patients and some first aid responders. You must never judge a patient's complaint based only on his or her appearance or physical condition. You must treat all abdominal emergencies as serious until proven otherwise.

The abdominal region contains several vital organs. They include the liver, stomach, colon, pancreas, spleen, and kidneys. While each of these organs has a specific set of signs and symptoms when injured or nonfunctional, it is necessary that you know only the general signs and symptoms of abdominal emergencies.

Learning Objectives

- Recognize the general signs and symptoms of abdominal emergencies.

- Demonstrate the appropriate treatment steps in emergency care for abdominal emergencies.

- Demonstrate the proper care for exposed abdominal organs.

ABDOMINAL EMERGENCIES: DANGER SIGNALS

When treating any female of childbearing age who complains of a sudden onset of abdominal pain, you must immediately activate the EMS system. The patient could have a tubal pregnancy. This can be a life-threatening emergency. It must be treated immediately.

Massive internal bleeding can occur within the abdomen before any signs or symptoms of shock appear. Always suspect internal bleeding. Immediately activate the EMS system.

Do not allow any patient with an abdominal emergency to eat or drink fluids. The patient may require surgery, and his or her stomach should be empty.

When treating a patient with exposed abdominal organs, never attempt to place the organs back in the abdominal cavity. Rather, cover them with a clean, moist cloth. Then treat the patient for shock, administer oxygen, monitor the patient's ABCH, and activate the EMS system.

ABDOMINAL EMERGENCIES: SIGNS AND SYMPTOMS

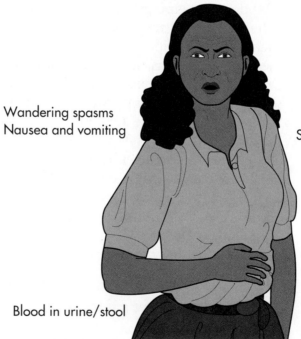

Wandering spasms
Nausea and vomiting

Shallow, rapid breathing

Tenderness
Abdominal rigidity
Severe pain
Soft-tissue injury
    with exposed
    organs

Blood in urine/stool

STEPS

TREATMENT OF ABDOMINAL EMERGENCIES

1.

2.

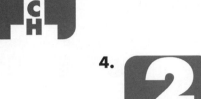

3. Be sure to control any massive external bleeding that you find.

4.

5.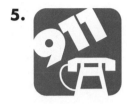

6.

7.

8. If necessary, treat the patient for shock.

REAL-LIFE RESPONSE

Your 30-year-old secretary approaches you and says that she is experiencing sudden abdominal pain. She lies down on the break room couch with her legs curled up to her chest. When you question her, she denies any significant medical history. She tells you she is feeling sick and begins to lose consciousness. A female employee tells you that the patient was complaining of massive vaginal bleeding earlier. Describe your emergency action plan.

EMERGENCY ACTION PLAN

_____

_____

_____

_____

_____

_____

_____

_____

CHAPTER 21

STROKE

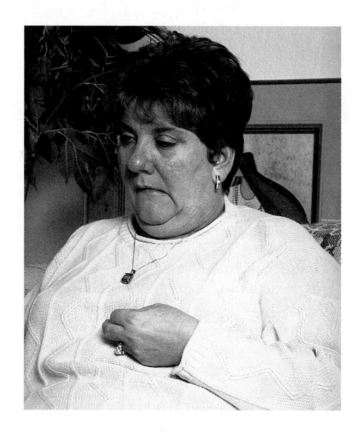

SYMBOL INDEX

Scene Safety

Body Substance Isolation

Activation of EMS

Initial Assessment

Ongoing Assessment

Rescue Breathing and Artificial Ventilation

Cardiopulmonary Resuscitation

Shock

Soft-Tissue Care

Musculoskeletal Care

Spinal Precautions

Oxygen Application

INTRODUCTION

Strokes occur when the blood's circulation to or within the brain is disrupted. Strokes are usually caused by blood clots, although they may occasionally be caused by hemorrhaging or tumors. Patients with high blood pressure, diabetes, and heart disease are most likely to suffer strokes.

Many patients will suffer strokelike attacks days or weeks before an actual stroke. These are called *transient ischemic attacks* (TIAs). TIAs usually last less than 24 hours. A history of frequent falls or unexplained soft-tissue injuries may be clues to earlier TIAs.

As a first aid responder, you should not attempt to distinguish between TIAs and complete strokes. When treating any patient who has signs and symptoms of a stroke, you should focus on managing any life-threatening complications the stroke may have caused. Maintaining an open and clear airway is your primary treatment consideration. Following that, you must immediately activate the EMS system. Getting the patient to the hospital quickly is extremely critical. The time from when a patient suffers a stroke to the time he or she receives treatment is directly related to the length of time the patient is in rehabilitation.

Although many stroke patients are unable to communicate and seem unable to hear, be very careful about what you say around them. In some cases, these patients are unable to express themselves but are able to understand what you say. Your words can have a major effect on how they react to your treatment.

Also be careful when moving a stroke patient who is unable to talk. You could cause the patient pain or injury and not even realize it.

Learning Objectives

- Recognize the signs and symptoms of strokes.

- Describe and demonstrate the proper emergency care for a patient suffering a stroke.

STROKE: DANGER SIGNALS

A sudden change in a patient's level of consciousness and accompanying paralysis often precede a loss of airway control. Be prepared to maintain the airway.

STROKE: SIGNS AND SYMPTOMS

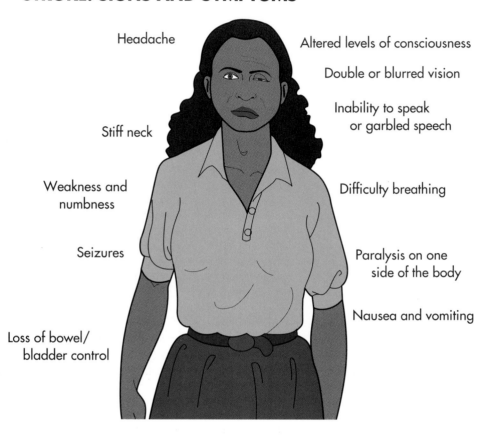

Headache

Altered levels of consciousness

Double or blurred vision

Inability to speak or garbled speech

Stiff neck

Weakness and numbness

Difficulty breathing

Seizures

Paralysis on one side of the body

Nausea and vomiting

Loss of bowel/ bladder control

STEPS

TREATMENT OF STROKE

1.

2.

3.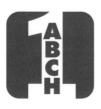

4.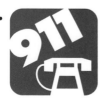

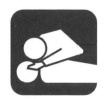

5. If necessary, deliver artificial ventilations to the patient.

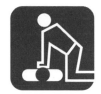

6. If necessary, perform CPR.

7.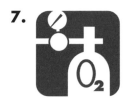

8.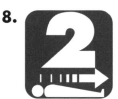

REAL-LIFE RESPONSE

You are visiting your best friend at her home when a neighbor knocks on the door. She tells you that she has been trying to get another neighbor to answer the door but has gotten no response. When you go to the neighbor's house, you see an elderly woman sitting on a couch. She seems unable to move. After entering the woman's home, you see that she is conscious. She slowly responds to your questions. She is confused and is having difficulty speaking. She has obvious facial paralysis on the left side of her body. Describe your emergency action plan.

EMERGENCY ACTION PLAN

_____

_____

_____

_____

_____

_____

_____

_____

_____

CHAPTER 22

DIABETIC EMERGENCIES

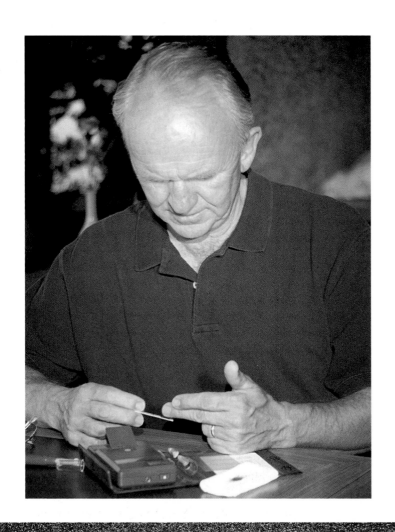

INTRODUCTION

Diabetes is a disease that affects the body's production and use of *insulin*. Insulin is a hormone that controls the amount of sugar found in the bloodstream.

Sugar is critical to the human body because the brain needs it in the proper amounts to function correctly. When too much or too little insulin is released into the bloodstream, the amount of sugar is altered. This in turn affects the brain's function. If this cycle is not corrected, changes in the brain's function can have tragic results. In the majority of cases, your quick action can save the diabetic patient's life.

There are two basic types of diabetic emergencies: *diabetic coma* and *insulin shock*. Diabetic coma is caused by *hyperglycemia*, or high blood sugar. A diabetic coma is associated with a slow onset of signs and symptoms. It is often caused by low levels of insulin. These patients require in-hospital observation to properly adjust their insulin levels.

Insulin shock is caused by *hypoglycemia*, or low blood sugar. Insulin shock is associated with a very sudden onset of signs and symptoms. It occurs when the patient has too much insulin in the bloodstream. This causes a rapid drop in the patient's blood sugar level. Most diabetics in this condition will rapidly lose consciousness. If you are called on to treat a person having a diabetic emergency, it will likely be insulin shock.

It is not important that you are able to distinguish between these two types of diabetic emergencies. However, it is important that you are able to recognize when a diabetic patient is having a serious emergency. You must also be able to deliver proper care prior to the arrival of the EMS responders.

People can become diabetic early in childhood. This is called juvenile-onset diabetes. The patient is usually insulin-dependent. People can also become diabetic as adults. This is called adult-onset diabetes. In some adult-onset diabetes patients, the condition can be controlled by diet. Others are insulin-dependent.

Learning Objectives

- Recognize the signs and symptoms of diabetic emergencies.

- Demonstrate an ability to assess and correctly treat the patient suffering a diabetic emergency.

DIABETES: DANGER SIGNALS

Diabetic emergencies are usually caused by insulin shock. Insulin shock has a very sudden onset and can kill a patient in a matter of minutes. When treating any patient experiencing a diabetic emergency, you must activate the EMS system immediately.

The diabetic patient can experience seizures. Be prepared to protect the patient's airway and deliver oxygen.

When delivering care to an unconscious patient, always look for medical alert medallions. They can give you valuable clues about the patient's medical problem.

DIABETES: SIGNS AND SYMPTOMS

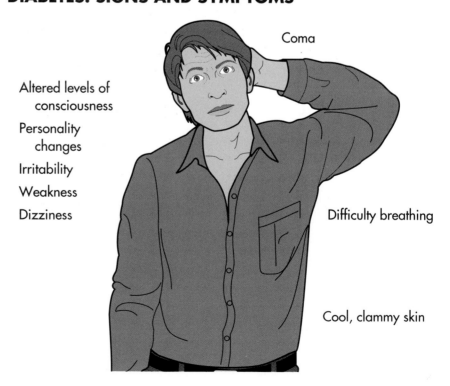

Coma

Altered levels of consciousness

Personality changes

Irritability

Weakness

Dizziness

Difficulty breathing

Cool, clammy skin

STEPS

TREATMENT OF DIABETIC EMERGENCIES

1.
2.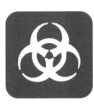
3.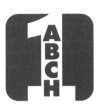
4.
5.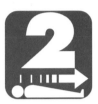
6.

7. If the patient is conscious and able to swallow, have him or her eat sugar. This can be in the form of syrup, jelly, juice, honey, apple sauce, or crushed sugar cubes.

8. Never give a semi-conscious patient anything by mouth. Wait for the EMS responders to arrive.

REAL-LIFE RESPONSE

As the supervisor of a group of farm workers, you notice that one employee has stopped working and is sitting in the shade. Other workers have told you that the man has some sort of medical condition that affects his sugar level. The patient appears to be about 18 years old. He complains of being very tired and says he wants to rest for a few minutes. The patient falls asleep as you talk with him. Describe your emergency action plan.

EMERGENCY ACTION PLAN

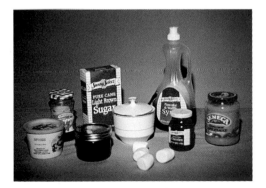

Different types of sugars can be given to a person suffering a diabetic emergency.

C H A P T E R 23

POISONING
AND OVERDOSE

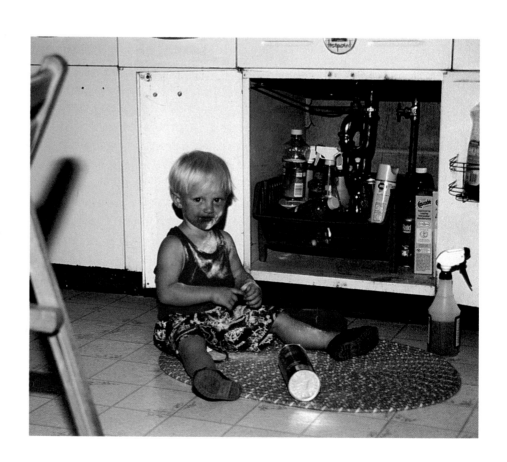

SYMBOL INDEX

Scene Safety

Body Substance Isolation

Activation of EMS

Initial Assessment

Ongoing Assessment

Rescue Breathing and Artificial Ventilation

Cardiopulmonary Resuscitation

Shock

Soft-Tissue Care

Musculoskeletal Care

Spinal Precautions

Oxygen Application

INTRODUCTION

Chemicals and other toxic substances are found in almost every occupational setting and in every home. Occasionally, these substances will poison a person. Poisons can enter the body through ingestion, inhalation, absorption, or injection. They can also enter the body through any combination of these ways.

Poisonings can be accidental or intentional. When intentional, they are usually a suicide attempt. In cases of intentional ingestions, people may attempt to poison themselves with toxic chemicals. They may also attempt to overdose on alcohol and other drugs.

Hazardous materials are another potential source of poisoning. In fact, as hazardous materials become more common, the chances of being poisoned by them increase. Unfortunately, accidents do occur, and if hazardous materials are involved, large-scale problems can result. If your workplace uses or produces hazardous materials, become familiar with your emergency response plan related to these materials. Review this plan often with your fellow first aid responders. During safety meetings or first-aid skills practice, use a hazardous materials spill as one type of practice scenario.

Regardless of whether they are accidental or intentional, all poisonings and overdoses are treated the same way at the first aid responder level. When treating any poisoning or overdose patient, you must pay close attention to the initial assessment. The status of the patient's ABCH can deteriorate quickly.

After you do the initial assessment, attempt to gather as much information about the substance as quickly as possible. Ask the patient or any bystanders what was ingested, when it was ingested, and approximately how much was ingested. Be prepared to relate this information to the responding EMS team. If time allows, attempt to locate the poison container to give to the EMS team.

You may also want to contact your local poison control center for additional information about how to treat your patient. These centers specialize in poisonings and overdoses. They are so useful, in fact, that most EMS professionals will call them as soon as they arrive on scene. Find out the phone number of your closest poison control center. Post the number near every phone in your workplace.

Learning Objectives

■ Demonstrate how to access and use the local poison control center.

■ Recognize the signs and symptoms of poisoning emergencies.

■ Demonstrate the proper emergency care for poisonings.

POISONING AND OVERDOSE: DANGER SIGNALS

Remember to perform a scene survey. Inhalation and absorption poisonings can cause serious injury. Do not enter the scene unless it is safe.

Patients who intentionally poison themselves often mix multiple substances. This can cause their condition to worsen very quickly. Concentrate on maintaining the patient's ABCH in all poisoning emergencies.

Many patients who have intentionally poisoned themselves will not give you an accurate history of the event. Never wait to activate the EMS system as you wait for the patient to tell you the truth.

Patients who have overdosed or been poisoned can become angry or hostile. If a patient does become hostile, make sure other first aid responders are with you as you treat the patient. If the situation becomes unsafe, leave immediately, and contact the police.

POISONING AND OVERDOSE: SIGNS AND SYMPTOMS

Altered levels of consciousness

Hallucinations

Burning sensation in the chest and throat

Headache

Excessive sweating

Burns/stains around the mouth

Difficulty breathing

Nausea/vomiting

Severe abdominal cramping

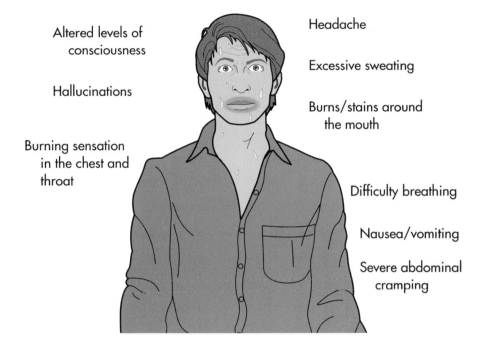

STEPS

TREATMENT OF POISONING AND OVERDOSE

1.

2.

3.

4.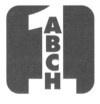

5. If necessary, deliver artificial ventilations to the patient.

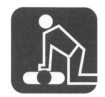

6. If necessary, perform CPR.

7.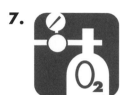

8.

REAL-LIFE RESPONSE

A woman pounds on your door, screaming. You open the door and see a neighbor holding her 2-year-old son in her arms. The woman says she knows that you run a day care center in your home. She asks you to help her son. As you question the woman, you determine that the boy possibly ingested several different liquid cleaners. The boy is covered with cleaner and has a strong odor of chemicals on his breath. Describe your emergency action plan.

EMERGENCY ACTION PLAN

_____

_____

_____

_____

_____

_____

_____

_____

_____

_____

_____

_____

_____

CHAPTER 24

SEIZURES, CONVULSIONS, AND ALTERED MENTAL STATUS

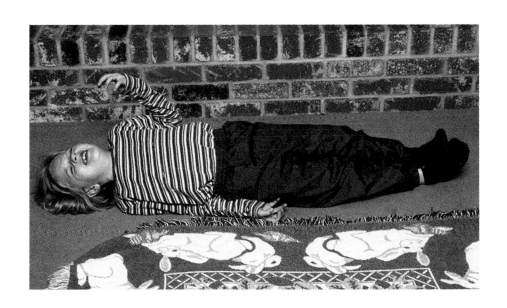

Scene Safety

 Body Substance Isolation

 Activation of EMS

 Initial Assessment

 Ongoing Assessment

 Rescue Breathing and Artificial Ventilation

 Cardiopulmonary Resuscitation

 Shock

 Soft-Tissue Care

 Musculoskeletal Care

 Spinal Precautions

 Oxygen Application

INTRODUCTION

Seizures—also known as convulsions—occur when the brain becomes extremely agitated and begins sending electrical stimuli to all of the body's muscles at the same time. This causes the body to shake and move violently.

There are several different causes of seizures. They include alcohol withdrawal, epilepsy, insulin reactions, overdoses, trauma, infections, and psychological disturbances. Seizure patients are usually aware of their condition and take medication to control the seizures. When you encounter any patient who is suffering a seizure, always look for medical alert medallions. They can give you valuable clues about the cause of the patient's seizures.

Most seizures last only a few minutes. They usually stop on their own. In rare cases, the patient may continue to have seizures for several minutes. Continuous seizure activity that lasts for several minutes is life-threatening. **Early activation of the EMS system is critical**.

People often have seizures in public places or at work. They are typically very confused immediately after the seizure and may react with anger, embarrassment, or fright. As a first aid responder, you should take appropriate measures to protect the patient from onlookers. You must also speak slowly and softly so as not to alarm or embarrass the patient.

Infants and young children often have seizures that are caused by fever. These are known as *febrile seizures*. They usually last only a minute or two. While febrile seizures are common, you must never assume that fever is the only cause of the seizure. Be sure to question family members or bystanders to try to determine if there might be another cause.

When delivering care to an infant or child who is experiencing seizures and you suspect that fever is the cause, immediately begin to cool the patient. You must be careful not to make the child too cold too rapidly, however. Cool the child just enough to return his or her body to a normal temperature. You can usually do this by placing a cold cloth under the armpits or across the abdomen or head. Then turn your attention back to managing the child's ABCH.

Learning Objectives

- Understand the various causes of seizures.

- Understand and demonstrate the proper emergency care for the seizure patient who has stopped seizing.

- Demonstrate the proper care for the patient who continues to seize without interruption.

- Demonstrate the correct care for an infant or child with a fever who has stopped seizing.

SEIZURES AND CONVULSIONS: DANGER SIGNALS

Never attempt to place anything in a seizure patient's mouth.

Monitor the seizure patient's airway for blood, vomit, and foreign objects during and after the seizure.

When treating any seizure patient, always make sure the airway is not blocked.

Any seizure that lasts for more than one or two minutes places the patient in extreme danger. If you are delivering care to a patient who has been seizing for longer than one or two minutes, time the length of the seizure activity. Then make sure that the EMS responders are on their way. If time allows, you can update the EMS responders and let them know the patient's status.

Never allow an infant or child to stay at home or at school following a seizure. He or she must be evaluated by a physician.

SEIZURES: SIGNS AND SYMPTOMS

PRE-SEIZURE

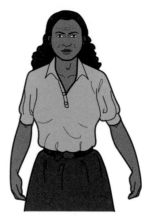

Hallucinations

Metallic taste in mouth

Abdominal pain

Twitching

DURING THE SEIZURE

Alternating contractions
of the muscles

No breathing

Unconsciousness
Eyes appear to roll back

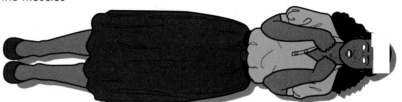

Violent jerking motions
Loss of bladder and bowel
control

Muscle rigidity

Frothing at the
mouth, clenched
teeth

AFTER THE SEIZURE

Deep breathing, then shallow,
irregular breaths

Small muscle twitching

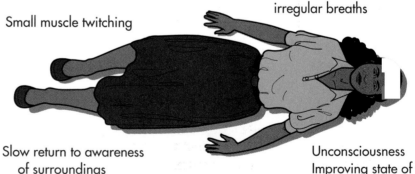

Slow return to awareness
of surroundings

Unconsciousness
Improving state of
consciousness

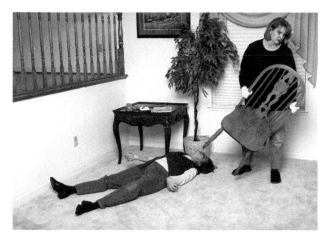

Moving any objects that could injure the patient during seizures.

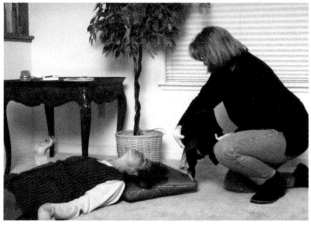

Placing a pillow under the patient's head.

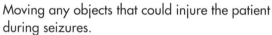

STEPS

TREATMENT OF SEIZURES

1.   **2.**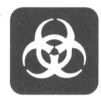

3. Clear the area of any hazards that could injure the patient.

4.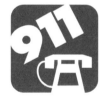

5. Perform an initial assessment after the seizures have stopped.

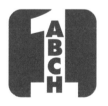

6. Place a pillow or other soft material under the patient's head. This is done to protect the patient's head from injury. Make absolutely sure the airway remains clear.

7.   **8.**   **9.**

REAL-LIFE RESPONSE

You are speaking with a co-worker when the woman suddenly stops talking and begins to look sick. As you question her, she slumps to the carpet. Her eyes begin to roll around, she shakes violently, and she makes an unusual sound. After about two minutes, you notice that she is bleeding slightly from her mouth and has stopped shaking. She rapidly falls asleep. You hear loud snoring sounds coming from her airway. Describe your emergency action plan.

EMERGENCY ACTION PLAN

_____

_____

_____

_____

_____

_____

_____

_____

_____

_____

_____

CHAPTER 25

ALLERGIC REACTIONS

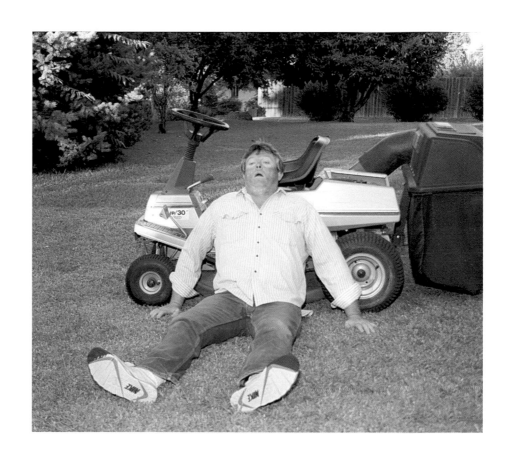

Scene Safety

Body Substance Isolation

Activation of EMS

Initial Assessment

Ongoing Assessment

Rescue Breathing and Artificial Ventilation

Cardiopulmonary Resuscitation

Shock

Soft-Tissue Care

Musculoskeletal Care

Spinal Precautions

Oxygen Application

INTRODUCTION

Allergies occur when the body comes into contact with certain proteins that it considers dangerous. The body's defense systems attack the protein with antibodies in an effort to kill it. In severe cases, the body's defense systems begin a dangerous cycle as they continue to try to kill the protein to protect the body. If this cycle is not stopped, the patient can die.

These severe allergic reactions can be caused by just about anything. Some of the more common causes are bee stings, dairy products, nuts, antibiotic medications, pollen, and shellfish. When a patient's allergic reaction is severe enough to cause the circulatory system to malfunction, *anaphylactic shock* begins. **Anaphylactic shock is life-threatening**. A patient can die within minutes if he or she is not treated immediately.

Most people who are allergic to something will have multiple exposures to the agent with an increasingly negative reaction. However, in rare cases, the patient can have a life-threatening allergic reaction during the first known exposure.

Learning Objectives

- Recognize the signs and symptoms of a severe allergic reaction.

- Demonstrate the emergency care to be provided for anaphylactic shock.

- Demonstrate the proper technique for removing a bee stinger.

ALLERGIC REACTIONS: DANGER SIGNALS

Severe allergic reactions are a life-threatening emergency. This is particularly true if anaphylactic shock occurs. These types of reactions can have a very rapid onset. You must begin treatment immediately. If the patient has even slight pain or discomfort, quickly activate the EMS system.

If a patient is suffering an allergic reaction, his or her airway can rapidly swell shut. Make sure you closely monitor and assist the patient's breathing if necessary. Never stick anything in the patient's mouth to look for swelling or damage.

ALLERGIC REACTIONS AND ANAPHYLACTIC SHOCK: SIGNS AND SYMPTOMS

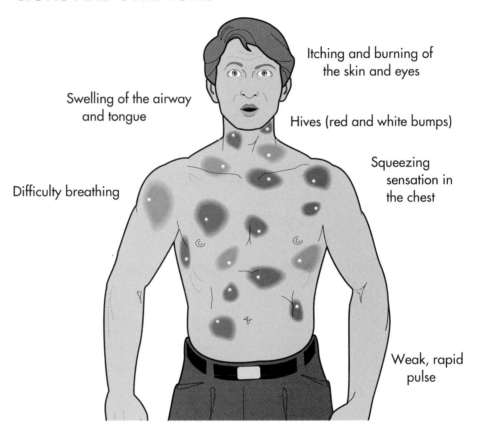

Itching and burning of the skin and eyes

Swelling of the airway and tongue

Hives (red and white bumps)

Difficulty breathing

Squeezing sensation in the chest

Weak, rapid pulse

 **STEPS**

TREATMENT OF SEVERE ALLERGIC REACTIONS

1. Make sure the agent that caused the allergic reaction is not present or is not a threat to you.

2.

3.

4.

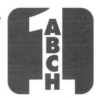

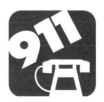

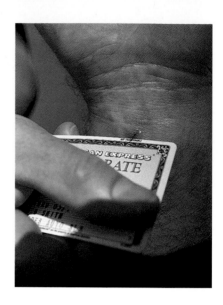

Removing a stinger using a credit card.

 **5.** If necessary, deliver artificial ventilations to the patient.

 6. If necessary, perform CPR.

7. 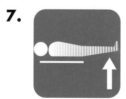   **8.** 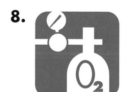   **9.**

10. If the person has been stung by a bee or wasp and the stinger is still in place, attempt to remove it. Use something with a strong edge, such as a credit card, to scrape across the skin and stinger. If you cannot find anything to use to scrape the stinger, pluck it out as quickly as possible.

11. Most people who have a tendency to experience allergic reactions usually carry allergy medication kits. If you are delivering care to a patient who has such a kit, help the patient locate the kit. If necessary, help the patient administer the medication.

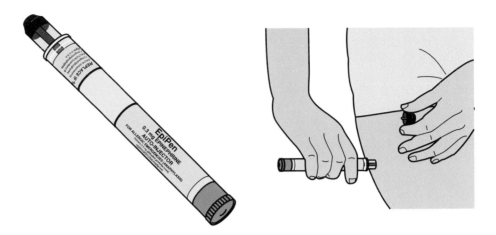

The EpiPen® is self-administered to treat severe allergic reactions.

REAL-LIFE RESPONSE

Your next-door neighbor comes running over to your house and screams that her husband has been stung by a bee and is having a terrible reaction. As you approach the scene, you note that the man appears to be about 45 years old. He is complaining of chest tightness, facial swelling, and itching. You notice that his lips, gums, and fingernails are turning blue. Describe your emergency action plan.

EMERGENCY ACTION PLAN

_____

_____

_____

_____

_____

_____

_____

_____

_____

_____

_____

_____

GLOSSARY

ABCH Assessment Process   This process consists of maintaining and treating the patient's airway, breathing, circulation, and hemorrhage. This process is the main component of the initial assessment.

Abdominal Distention   A condition that can occur when delivering artificial ventilations. When ventilations are delivered too forcefully, air can be forced into the stomach, causing it to become distended. Abdominal distention can prevent the lungs from expanding and filling properly.

Abrasion   A superficial soft-tissue injury in which the skin is scraped or scratched.

Airway Management   The process of ensuring that a patient's airway remains open and clear.

Amputation   Technically a soft-tissue injury, an amputation occurs when a body part is completely severed from the body.

Anaphylactic Shock   An extremely exaggerated and life-threatening allergic reaction.

Artificial Ventilations   A method of delivering air to a patient who is not breathing or who is breathing inadequately. For first aid responders, this is accomplished on adults by placing the mouth over the patient's mouth, pinching the patient's nose shut, and breathing into the patient's mouth. A pocket mask should be used whenever possible when delivering artificial ventilations. Also known as rescue breathing.

Automatic External Defibrillator   A device that can assess the need for, and automatically deliver, an electric shock to the heart in an attempt to restart it. Also known as an AED.

AVPU Scale   This scale is used to help determine a patient's level of consciousness. A = Alert; V = Responds to verbal stimuli; P = Responds only to painful stimuli; U = Unconscious/Unresponsive.

Avulsion   A soft-tissue injury in which the skin is either partially or completely torn from the body.

Barrier to Action   Any psychological response that prevents a person from delivering emergency care. Examples include a fear of blood, a fear of injuring the patient, and a fear of liability.

Body Substance Isolation Precautions   A standard of protection that treats all body fluids as potentially infectious. Previously known as universal precautions.

Brachial Pulse   The pulse found on the inside of a patient's arm at the elbow joint.

Bronchiolitis   Inflammation of the bronchioles, or small branches of the airway. Bronchiolitis is fairly common among infants and children under the age of 2 years.

Cardiac Arrest   A life-threatening condition in which the heart stops circulating blood or stops beating.

Cardiopulmonary Resuscitation   A technique of providing artificial ventilations and chest compressions to a patient who is not breathing and does not have a pulse. Also known as CPR.

Carotid Pulse   The pulse found on both sides of a patient's neck.

Chest Compressions   A technique used to restart a patient's heart during CPR. The emergency responder's hands are placed over the patient's sternum, compressing the chest wall.

Chief Complaint   A patient's main concern, medical condition, or primary reason for needing assistance.

Circulation   The process of delivering oxygenated blood to the body's tissues. A patient's circulation is checked by assessing the pulse.

Closed Fracture   An injury in which a bone is broken but does not pierce the skin.

Communicable/Infectious Disease   Any virus, bacteria or microorganism that can be transferred from one person to another.

Critical Incident Stress Management/Debriefing   A process in which counselors help emergency responders deal with the emotional and psychological stress associated with a traumatic event. Also known as CISMor CISD.

Croup   A virus that causes inflammation of various components of the airway. Croup is fairly common among infants and children.

Diabetic Coma   A coma that occurs in diabetic patients. It is caused by inadequate levels of insulin in the body.

Dislocation   An injury in which a bone is pushed or pulled from its joint.

DOTS   An acronym used to remember conditions to look for during the ongoing assessment. D = Deformities; O = Open injuries; T = Tenderness; S = Swelling.

Epiglottitis   A potentially life-threatening respiratory illness that involves inflammation of the epiglottis. It is most common among infants and children.

Febrile Seizures   Seizures caused by high fever. They typically occur in infants and children.

Femoral Pulse   The pulse found in a patient's groin.

Finger Sweep   A technique in which the finger is used to dislodge and remove a foreign object in an unconscious patient's mouth.

First-Degree Burn   A superficial burn that involves only the outer layer of the skin. It is the least serious of the three burn classifications.

Flail Chest   A condition in which multiple ribs are fractured in multiple places.

Foreign-Body Airway Obstruction   A condition in which a foreign object blocks the normal flow of oxygen in the airway. Also known as an FBAO.

Fracture   An injury involving a break in a bone.

Golden Hour   A premise that patients who are suffering from severe trauma have the best chance of survival if they can be delivered to an operating room within one hour of their injuries.

Good Samaritan Laws   Laws that are designed to offer protection for people who deliver voluntary emergency care.

Head-Tilt/Chin-Lift Maneuver   A technique used to open a patient's airway. One hand is used to tilt the patient's head back. The other is used to lift the patient's chin up and forward.

Heat Cramps   Painful muscle cramps resulting from excessive salt and water loss.

Heat Exhaustion   Weakness caused by excessive salt and water loss.

Heat Stroke   A life-threatening condition characterized by the complete inability to release heat from the body.

Heimlich Maneuver   A technique performed on a patient with a complete airway obstruction. Abdominal thrusts are used to expel the object.

Hemorrhage   Excessive, potentially life-threatening bleeding.

Hyperglycemia   A condition caused by increased levels of glucose, or blood sugar, in the bloodstream.

Hyperventilation   A type of breathing emergency in which the patient is breathing at an accelerated rate.

Hypoglycemia   A condition caused by low levels of glucose, or blood sugar, in the bloodstream.

Hypothermia   Decreased body temperature.

Immobilization   A technique that involves splinting an injured body part, such as a limb. This is done to protect the body part from further injury.

Impaled Object   A condition in which a foreign object is imbedded in the body.

Initial Assessment   The first assessment done on a patient. The purpose is to determine and treat any life-threatening conditions the patient might have. The main component of the initial assessment is maintenance and treatment of the patient's airway, breathing, circulation, and hemorrhage (ABCH).

Insulin   A hormone naturally produced in the body. It is also a manufactured medication used by many diabetics.

Insulin Shock   A type of shock that occurs in diabetic patients. It is caused by excessive levels of insulin in the body.

Jaw-Thrust Maneuver   A technique used to open a patient's airway in cases of suspected spine injury. The fingers are used to lift the patient's jaw up and forward without extending the neck or head.

Laceration   A soft-tissue injury in which the skin is torn or cut.

Laryngectomy   Surgical removal of the larynx.

Look, Listen, Feel   A method of assessing a patient's breathing. Look for chest movement; listen for breathing; and feel for air against the cheek and for the chest rising and falling.

Mechanism of Injury/Illness   Factors that are involved in or produce an injury or illness.

Musculoskeletal Injury   An injury that involves bones, joints, muscles, or tendons.

Occlusive Dressing   A dressing that creates an airtight seal over a wound.

Ongoing Assessment   A thorough, head-to-toe assessment of a patient. It is performed after the initial assessment to identify any conditions that might have been missed during the initial assessment. It is also used to monitor the patient's condition.

Open Fracture   An injury in which a broken bone pierces the skin. Previously known as a compound fracture.

Personal Protective Devices   Equipment used or worn to protect against injury and the spread of communicable diseases. Examples include an eye and face shield, disposable gloves, a gown, and a mask.

Pressure Points   Locations in the body where blood flow can be interrupted by applying direct pressure over an artery, compressing it against a bone.

Puncture Wound   A soft-tissue injury in which the skin is pierced.

Radial Pulse   The pulse found on the thumb side of a patient's wrist.

Recovery Position   A side-lying position that helps protect a patient's airway.

Rescue Breathing   See *artificial ventilations*.

RICE   An acronym used to remember the process for treating a muscle or bone injury that does not involve exposed bone ends. R = Rest; I = Ice; C = Compression; E = Elevation.

SAMPLE   An acronym used to remember the type of information gathered when taking a patient's history. S = Signs and symptoms; A = Allergies; M = Medications; P = Pertinent past history; L = Last oral intake; E = Events that might have caused the injury or illness.

Scope of Practice   The care and treatment that an emergency responder is legally allowed to deliver.

Second-Degree Burn   A moderate-severity burn in which the first layer of skin is completely burned and the second layer is damaged. It is the second most serious of the three burn classifications.

Shock   A condition caused by inadequate amounts of oxygen being delivered to the body's cells.

Shortness of Breath   A condition in which a patient is experiencing difficulty breathing.

Signs and Symptoms   A way of determining any conditions a patient might have. Signs are conditions that the patient displays; symptoms are conditions that the patient describes.

Sprain   An injury to a ligament that causes pain and disability.

Stoma   A permanent surgical opening in the neck and throat through which a person breathes. Typically performed in people who have had a laryngectomy.

Strain   An injury to a muscle and its surrounding tendons that causes pain and disability.

Sucking Chest Wound   A life-threatening condition in which an open chest wound draws air into the chest cavity.

Sudden Infant Death Syndrome   The sudden, unexplained death of an infant or young child. The death usually occurs when the child is asleep. Also known as SIDS.

Third-Degree Burn   A high-severity burn in which all layers of the skin are damaged. It is the most serious of the three burn classifications.

Transient Ischemic Attack   Also known as a TIA, a transient ischemic attack is a recurrent episode of neurological deficit that is similar to a stroke. Many patients will suffer a TIA days or weeks before an actual stroke. TIAs usually last less than 24 hours.

Triage   A system of assessing and categorizing multiple patients according to the severity of their illnesses or injuries.

Xiphoid Process   The spot in the chest where the ribs join.

INDEX